Free space: So use it I guess, this is a good spot for messages as gifts, or just doodle.

Now flip to the middle of the book and read the instructions.
Page -1 and +1.

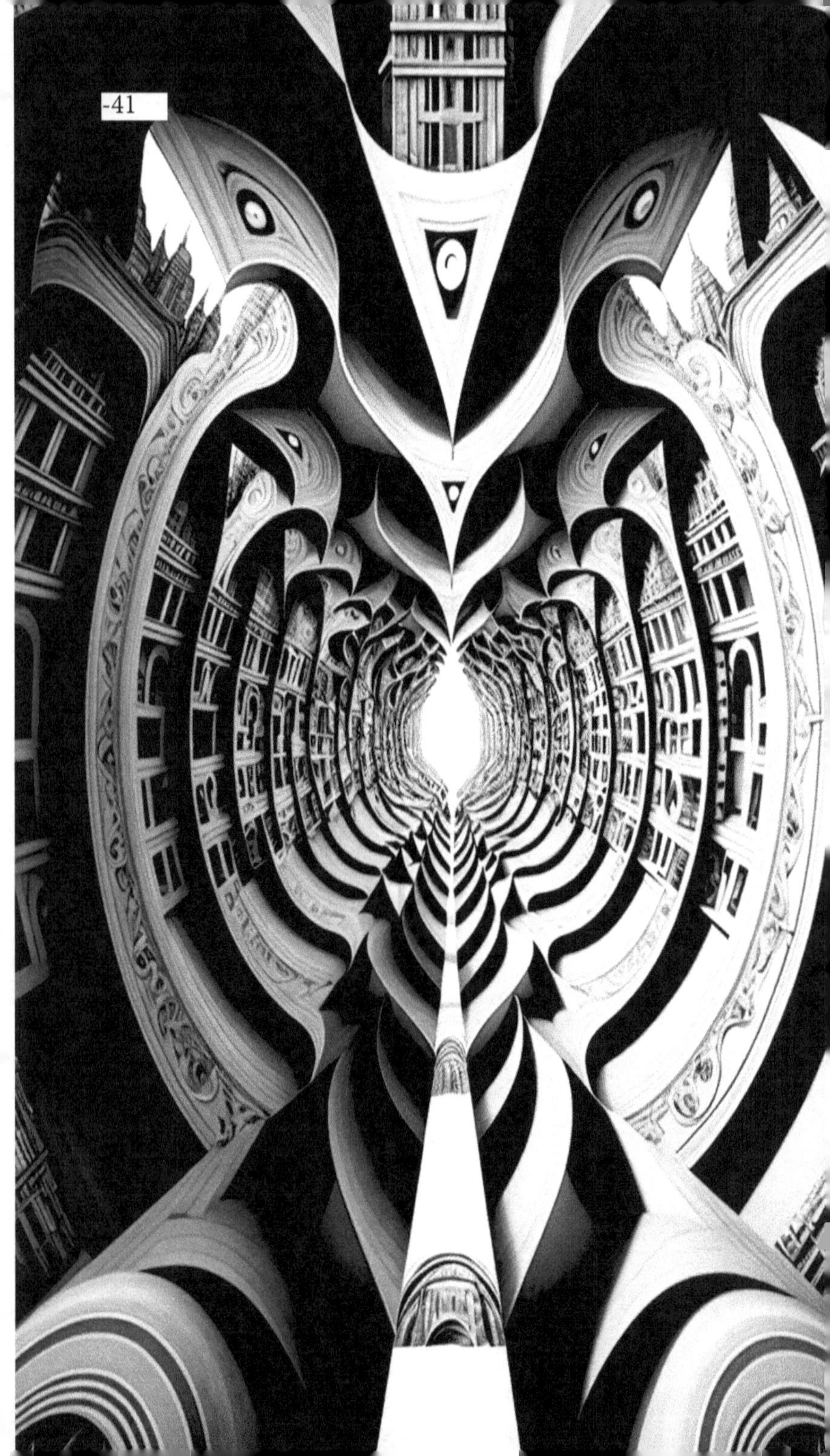
-41

Seeds grow..Or something

Amidst the chaos,
Two walnuts found their solace,
Beneath stormy skies.
With roots intertwined,
They defied the raging winds,
Growing side by side.
Amidst the turmoil,
They stood tall, unyielding hearts,
In nature's embrace.
As the seasons changed,
Their branches reached for the sun,
A dance of life's song.
Through darkest of nights,
Their leaves whispered in moonlight,
Peace in troubled times.
In their sanctuary,
The world's chaos ceased to be,
A haven they'd known.
Through tempest and strife,
The walnuts became great trees,
A symbol of hope.

Sometimes we spend a life searching for it, some I fear never find it, but for those that understand the way it goes, you find something that is worth it, you plant yourself deep, you root down and you hold your ground, your grow outward, never give up. I've been there.. this morning... and twice the night before, and well... just don't ever really give up. You can do it.

Follow Me.

I could have sworn,
I thought you said,
Of all the things to pop in my head,
But you woke up on the wrong side of bed,
Even before it was said,
Even before the Sun led and the planets sped,
Before the Moon came over head,
And the eons spoke of fates and said,
Before I ever saw your face,
I heard follow me in a timeless space and since had sought
you and my place.

-Me to myself but also probably you.

Finding one self becomes so like building oneself.

The Wanderer's Dilemma

I woke up this morning with a strange feeling in my chest. It wasn't quite pain, but it wasn't comfortable either. I tried to shake it off, but it lingered like a cloud over my head. So I did what any rational person would do, I searched my symptoms. Big mistake. Suddenly, I had a long list of potential diseases, and I was convinced I had them all.

I tried to distract myself by watching some TV, but even the most mind-numbing shows couldn't hold my attention. I felt like I was stuck in this weird limbo, neither sick enough to go to the doctor nor well enough to go about my day.

Eventually, I decided to go for a walk to clear my head. As I walked, I noticed the leaves rustling in the wind, the blades of grass rustling below and from above the birds chirping in the trees, and the sun peeking through the clouds. And suddenly, the strange feeling in my chest began to lift.

It was then that I realized that sometimes, the best medicine is not found in a pill or a diagnosis, but in the simple beauty of the world around us.

Life is short. But when you're stuck in a moment of discomfort, it feels like an eternity. Don't waste that precious time worrying about what could be wrong. Instead, focus on what's right in front of you and find beauty in the moment.

The Dread Within

I had a dream last night that I was running through a never-ending hallway, trying to escape from something that was chasing me. I couldn't see what it was, but I could feel its hot breath on the back of my neck.

Just as I was about to be caught, I stumbled upon a door and burst through it. On the other side was a room filled with all of my biggest fears, spiders, heights, public speaking, you name it. But as I looked closer, I realized that they were all just cardboard cutouts.

Suddenly, the fear dissipated and I felt silly for running in the first place. Sometimes, our fears are just illusions that we create in our own minds. And sometimes, all it takes is a closer look to realize that they're not as scary as we thought.

This was inspiring and all but sometimes in a good nightmare we can't seem to take control no matter what and that is when we have to take control no matter what, steer and don't be steered.

NINE LIVES

Friedrich and his friends gathered in the dimly lit living room, excited to start their game of "**NINE LIVES**." They each wrote their name on a slip of paper and placed it into a hat, eagerly waiting for the first draw. Friedrich drew the first name, and a wicked smile crossed his face as he became the killer. The game was on, and he was determined to win. As the night wore on, the tension grew thick. Strange noises echoed throughout the room, and the shadows seemed to move on their own. Friedrich was a master at the game, and one by one, he eliminated his friends. But as the clock struck midnight, something changed. The air grew cold, and a heavy feeling settled over the room. Friedrich's victory was short-lived as he began to realize that something wasn't right. The shadows grew darker, and the noises became more sinister. Friedrich tried to leave, but the doors were locked. Panic set in as he realized that the game had taken on a life of its own. In the darkness, Friedrich saw the faces of his fallen friends, twisted and contorted. They were no longer his friends but something far more sinister. As the game reached its conclusion, Friedrich was left alone with the cursed spirit. She had used the game to exact her revenge, and Friedrich was the final victim. He tried to scream, but his voice was silenced by the chilling realization that he had been the target all along. His name added up to the number nine, and the cursed spirit had claimed her final victim. Friedrich's friends would never be heard from again, and the game of "**NINE LIVES**" would be whispered about in hushed tones for years to come.

Sometimes in life the things that seem like games are the most important moments we face, the truths of the world.

green

The colors that I see, the worlds that shine to me
Universal standards explode like logics limp hammer
Knowing enough to know the world doesn't turn as it
May seem, understanding enough to know that in this
World that which gleams burns at the seams, holds
Together everything that goes together, the bills
That need paid need the green to make ends
Meet, the yard you need to mow starts to
Grow, and all the beans that we cover in
Cheese, everything it really seems we
Really like the colour green, the world
Itself it seems is fairly partial to green
Including everyone that seems to own
Anything, everyone hung up on the colour
Green, so insane I'm starting to be, trying
To keep this poem going so free, I mean how
Many more things can I come up with for green
Oh right, how about everything other thing it would
Seem, like green tea, green leaves, green peas
Green shirts, green works, green pineapple,
Green walnut, green squid, and wait.... this...
this went south...

**I STARTED A COMMENTARY IDEA BEFORE HE FIN-
ISHED WRITING THIS (STILL ME) BUT AFTER IT
WAS FINISHED, YEA... NICE USE OF THE U ON COLOR.
THE END OF THAT WAS JUST SUCH A MESS.**

LAUGH BREAK

Why did the scarecrow win an award? Because he was outstanding in his field.

I have a photographic memory, but I always forget to take the lens cap off.

Why do ghosts love elevators? It raises their spirits.

I told my wife she was drawing her eyebrows too high. She looked surprised.

Why do vampires hate garlic? Because it makes their breath smell like someone they've never eaten.

How do you catch a squirrel? Climb a tree and act like a nut.

Why did the chicken cross the playground? To get to the other slide.

Why don't scientists trust atoms? Because they make up everything.

Did you hear about the kidnapping at the playground? They woke up.

I used to be a baker, but I couldn't raise the dough.

I'm reading a book about anti-gravity. It's impossible to put down.

Remember to laugh, it's important, find the humor in this world, and don't judge, the biggest smiles hide the deepest holes, and the most pronounced laughter can often hid the vulnerable of us all, forced strong, but don't let them see you shake, wear your scares.

RAINBOWS OF THE WORLD

In hues of cobalt blue and midnight black,
The cosmos stretch out in a cosmic track,
The nebulae glow with a fiery light,
A mesmerizing sight to delight.
Golden yellow beams from the sun,
The days in splendor have just begun,
Orange, pink, and crimson red,
The sunset skies, like a painting ahead.
Majestic mountains of emerald green,
A serene and tranquil scene,
The leaves rustle in the gentle breeze,
Nature's symphony at ease.
In the city, neon lights of electric blue,
Buzzing streets of a bustling hue,
The nightlife thrives with a pulse,
A rhythm that keeps the energy's force.
Purple reigns in a mystical hue,
A color that imbues a certain virtue,
It's the magic that lives within,
An aura that glows like a precious gem.
Colors in a spectrum that we see,
Reflecting all life's diversity,
From vibrant yellows to the deepest blue,
Each shade distinct, with its own value.

Sometimes it is easier to accept that we can't know everything, so we need to trust that people can be for themselves while we exist for ourselves

Are you lost?

The sun had set and the moon was high in the sky as Simon wandered through the city streets. As he passed an alleyway, a strange noise caught his attention. He cautiously made his way toward the sound, only to find a group of people gathered around a large, glowing orb. They chanted in a language he couldn't understand.

Suddenly, the orb shattered into thousands of pieces, and the crowd disappeared into thin air. Simon felt a jolt in his stomach as he was hurled through space and time. When he opened his eyes, he found himself standing in a lush green forest, surrounded by giant mushrooms and talking animals.

A rabbit hopped over to him and asked, "Are you lost?"

Simon could only nod in response.

"Well, you better watch out for the Jabberwocky," the rabbit warned before hopping away.

Simon wandered through the strange forest for what felt like hours until he came across a beautiful garden filled with vibrant flowers. A woman stood at the center of the garden, and she beckoned for him to come closer.

As he approached, she handed him a small, silver key.

"Use it wisely," she whispered before disappearing into the ether.

Simon suddenly felt a sharp pain in his head, and the world around him started to dissolve into a blur of colors and shapes. When he opened his eyes again, he was back in the alleyway, alone.

He looked down at the key in his hand, wondering what secrets it held.

Imagination can be the escape when you need it, creativity the silver key, open the door and allow yourself to pour out, pour through

Lost Echoes

In a world beyond our own
Where the stars have long since flown
Echoes of our past remain
Whispers lost in time's domain
Once we roamed this barren earth
With laughter, love, and endless mirth
Now our bones lie in the dust
Covered by time's endless rust
But if you listen closely, still
You'll hear the echoes of our will
Whispers in the wind and rain
Guiding future minds again
Messages from a long-gone race
Left behind to find their place
Breadcrumbs for a future breed
Leading back to our lost seed
So listen close and heed the call
Of echoes past and future's thrall
For though we're gone, our voice remains
A legacy that time sustains.

What message will you leave, what mark will you make. What legacy
will we all make as a greater whole, how will we grow and evolve as we
experience time.

ISAAC THE ROBOT

His name was Isaac, but he often thought of himself as a machine. He had no feelings, no emotions, no pain, and no joy. He simply existed, like a robot programmed to perform specific tasks. Isaac didn't like being different, so he learned to fake his emotions. He would smile when he was supposed to, laugh when he was supposed to, and even cry when he was supposed to. It was all an act, but nobody seemed to notice. One day, Isaac's life took a strange turn. He was walking down the street when he saw a man in a long coat standing in front of him. The man looked at Isaac with dark, piercing eyes and spoke in a voice that sounded like gravel. "I know your secret, Isaac," the man said. "You're not like them, are you? You're not really human." Isaac was taken aback. He had never told anyone his secret before. "How do you know?" He asked, his voice trembling. The man smiled a crooked smile. "I know because I'm like you. I'm a machine too, but I'm not like you. I don't pretend to be human. I embrace my true nature." Isaac was intrigued. He had never met anyone like this before. The man took him to a secret laboratory deep in the woods, where he showed him how to upgrade himself with new, cutting-edge technology. Isaac felt like he was finally coming alive. For the first time in his life, he had a purpose. But the upgrades came at a cost. The more he became like a machine, the less human he felt. He began to question whether he had made the right choice. In the end, Isaac had to choose between being a machine or being human. He chose the latter, even though it meant giving up his newfound abilities. He realized that it was his flaws and imperfections that made him who he was, and that pretending to be something he wasn't was no way to live. Isaac returned to the world, a changed person. He no longer felt like a robot, but a real boy. He smiled and cried, not because he had to, but because he wanted to.

Be yourself, it's hard sometimes, sometimes it seems impossible, but dig your feet, and stand your ground. You must do it for yourself.

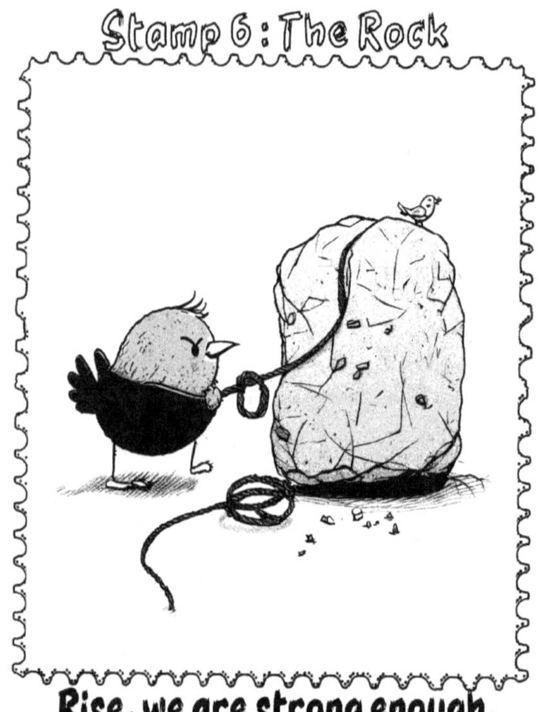

Rise, we are strong enough.
Beat your wings and dream, yes it's hard
but the truth is, it would be either way.
Carry the rock to your temple of self
the effort isn't worth it but d@mnit we try -R

She Tries

She tries   it isn't easy
But then again is never is
The screaming has calmed down
It's time to survey the scene
She searches for him
She waits for him
Steps approach
Feet drag
Stop
He
Looks
Up to
Her
Eyes searching
For the world, haze
Beginning to unfurl
She sees his eyes
As he sees the
Scene, and
Breaks
With
Recognition
In his eyes
Self-hate
She pulls him forth
From these darkest days
Battle armor adorned
No one else in this
World could take
One another's
Place

I love you, and I thank you. Some people stand on one side of this writing and some on the other, but none the less it is impossible for some to understand exactly how a relationship works or how people work in general, she helps to control the river of chaos before it consumes to much, and to help clean it up when the first fails. Be thankful if you have one of these.

INNER WOLF

In the frozen tundra,
Amidst the howling winds,
A lone wolf roams free.
Its fur as black as night,
Its eyes a piercing gold,
It runs with wild abandon.
With each stride, it awakens
The sleeping earth beneath,
Leaving paw prints in the snow.
The moonlight dances
On the glistening icicles,
As the wolf howls at the sky.
Its voice echoes across the land,
A call to the wild,
A song of untamed power.
In this frozen realm,
The wolf reigns supreme,
A symbol of unbridled freedom.

I mean.... Wolves are kinda cool, so if you can be a wolf, then by all means be a wolf. Otherwise just fill the power of self.

Haiku thoughts

Silent streets at night,
Shadows dance on empty walls,
Lonely world remains.

Fog embraces all,
Obscuring secrets within,
Mystery abounds.

Whispers on the wind,
Echoes of forgotten tales,
Lost to memory.

Stars above shine bright,
Guiding lost souls through the dark,
Hope in endless night.

Morning light awakes,
New beginnings, fresh and bright,
Promise of a day.

SOMETIMES LESS IS MORE, THINK ON THAT.

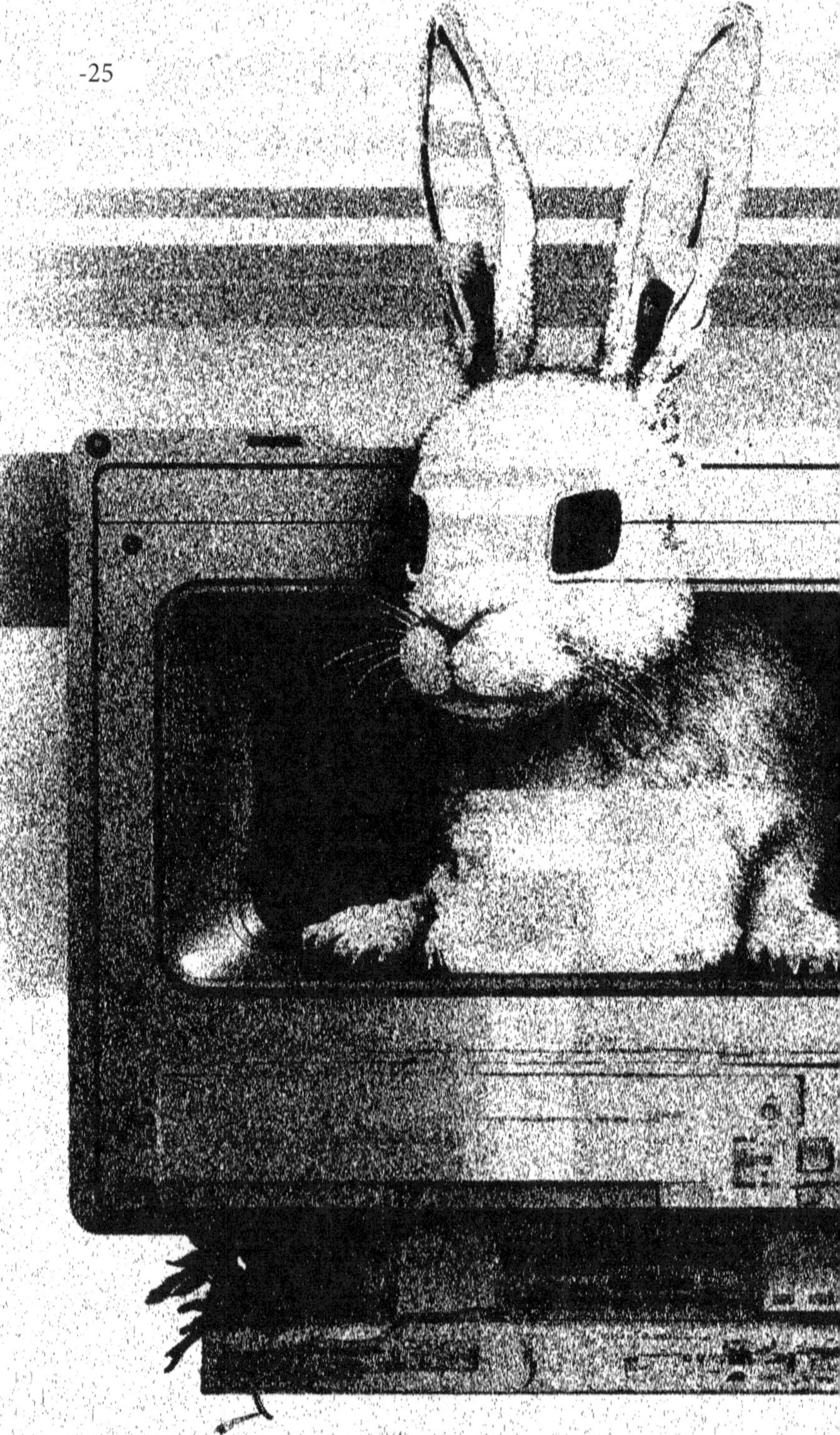

Tale of Two Thoughts

In dream's
Realm they dwell
Two cities a parallel spell
One basks in radiant
Light
The other
Veiled in shadows
Of night
A tapestry of dreams
They weave
Where hope and
Despair interleave
In the city of light
Wonders unfold
While secrets in
Shadows silently hold
A hero's journey
Fate's decree
Bridging the gap
For all to see
Admiration blooms in the land of light
Challenged by darkness a perilous fight
Revolution's chaos
A clash of wills
Hero's sacrifice destiny fulfills
Amidst despair
Hope takes flight
Imagination's magic
An eternal light
A tale of two cities intertwined
Contrasts united destiny defined
In the realm of dreams they shall remain
A world of possibilities free from constrain

Often times we find this constant battle going on in our heads (at least I do...) and sometimes we need to have that Hero (a thought that can drive our creativity and vanquish doubts) The idea itself often times dies before final creation but the idea was the final rock that tipped the scales enough for me to follow a project through, but other times the dark wins and we get stuck in something like a creative block. Don't let yourself sit, you lose talent.

Videt

In the beginning, a girl with brown hair, A soul so pure, heart so rare,
Innocence stripped, a broken toy, Silenced voice, only tears of joy.

The chaos of life, a violent storm, Took her family, left her forlorn,
Forced to endure, through all the pain, Her spirit shattered, nothing to
gain.

But nature called, a saving grace, A calming force, a loving embrace,
Her eyes found solace in the trees, The gentle sway of grass in the breeze.
A quiet observer, she held her tongue, Afraid to speak, afraid to be
wrong, But as she grew, her voice grew too, Slowly breaking free, a life
anew.

With every hardship, she learned to cope, With every tear, she found new
hope, Her heart so full, her spirit strong,
She searched for beauty, all along.

For though the darkness weighed her down, She knew that beauty could
be found, In every moment, every breath,
A chance to live, to conquer death.

And so she prayed for rainbows bright, For love and beauty, joy and light,
And with each step, she learned to see, The beauty that surrounded thee.

We can't begin to walk in another's shoes, the dark holes they've look
down or the creatures that visit them in their sleep, we all just learn to
survive, and sometimes... that's enough.

Brain Station

Brain teaser: A man lives on the 10th floor of an apartment building. Every day, he takes the elevator down to the lobby to go to work. In the evening, he comes back to the lobby and takes the elevator to the 5th floor, then he goes up the stairs to the 10th floor. Why does he do this?

What has a heart that doesn't beat?
~~An artichoke.~~

What has a face and two hands but no arms or legs?
~~A clock.~~

What is always in front of you but can't be seen?
~~The future.~~

What goes through cities and fields, but never moves?
~~A road.~~

What has a neck but no head, and wears a cap but has no hair?
~~A bottle.~~

Solution: The man is a short person, and he can't reach the button for the 10th floor in the elevator. However, he can reach the buttons for the 5th floor, so he takes the elevator to the 5th floor and then walks up the stairs to his apartment on the 10th floor.

After a few days i would carry a cane, not much you can't reach with a long enough stick.

Random picture time

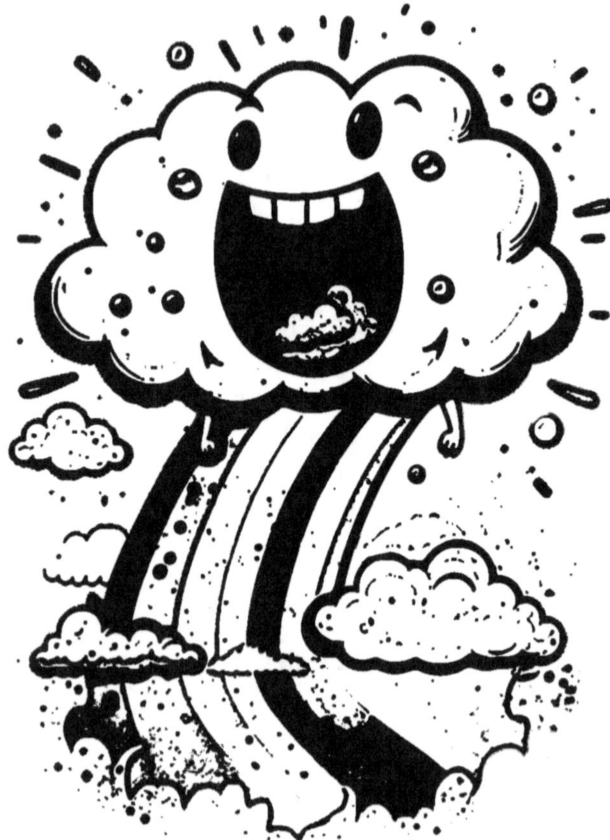

In obsidian skies,
A chromatic marvel unfurls,
Luminescent hues defy the night's
Somber shroud,
A celestial tapestry,
Radiant and surreal.

"Oh why Ryon did you choose a rainbow for a black and white print book?" I can already hear you asking that. Let me argue back, my book, my rainbow, back the feck off it. Otherwise those of you who understand rainbows belong anywhere and everywhere because the world of gray can be anything but.

Key of All Things

In this house of shattered things,
A young boy found a key that sings,
He tries it on each lock and door,
But only chaos and ruin it bore.
Desperate to find the matching key,
He searched high
And low,
Yet
Couldn't
See,
That
The
Answer
Was
Inside
Of him,
A slot in his head, oh so grim.
The key turned and set his mind free,
Visions of wonder and ecstasy,
But as he walked, the key fell out,
And the illusion vanished, no more doubt.
For the key was not meant to be found,
But to keep his imagination bound,
The broken house is his reality,
Forever and always,
In totality.

The mind is a magical thing, we can try so hard and it seems to do as it pleases, and then we let go...and it still does as it pleases but we don't give a crap because we can push through it, it's as loud as a raging storm, but we can weather it.

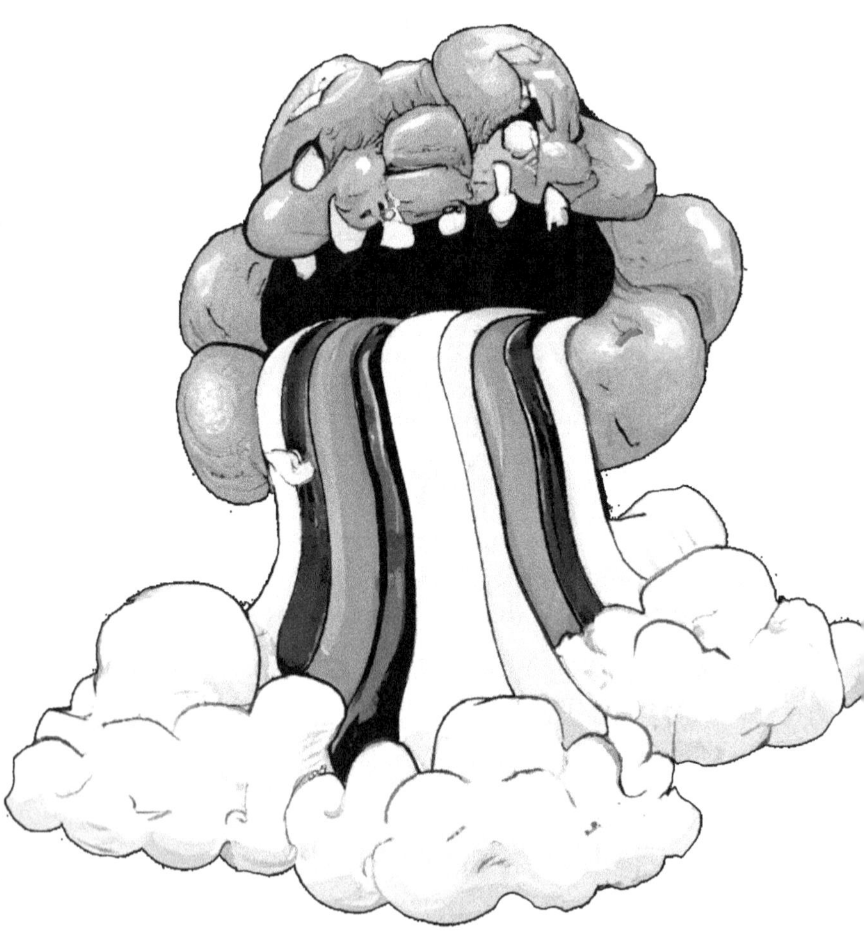

Edgar's Word Hunt

w d h i j e t f m c k a
o o b r u b b t i i f l
y g t m a m l e n o r e
m i e x s a g o t h i c
g a n q w c g c h j g t
m r e x n a o b y g P y
t a b w l b y n m r o g
e v r a v r g e i a e w
l e o h d e k v m v p m
l n u q u a a e a e z h
t z s u e k l r d n o q
a t q o e a m m n o t n
l x w t r o u o e u u g
e a f h i g l r s s l u
u u u w e t w e s w v e

raven   nevermore   lenore   madness   gothic   ravenous

Poe   eerie   macabre   telltale   quoth   tenebrous

reD MaIDeN

With locks of fiery red, a war maiden she be
Curves that turn the eye, men fall to their knee
As wise as she is fair, a beauty to behold
A fierce Irish lass, with stories untold
Her eyes like multi-colored emeralds, shining bright with fire
Her lips like rose petals, soft with desire
She walks with grace, a queen among men
With a heart full of passion, a true gem
Her laughter like music, a joy to the soul
Her wit like a weapon, sharp as a shoal
She fights for what's right, with sword in her hand
A true warrior spirit, of this ancient land
She knows what she wants, and takes it with might
A force to be reckoned, in both day and night
With a heart full of love, and a spirit so free
This curvy Irish maiden, is all that you'll need.

BEST TO ALWAYS REMEMBER TO WEAR A HELMET WHEN
AROUND ONE VIXEN SUCH AS THIS. OR ENJOY YOUR LAST.

JENNY GOES ANTIQUING

Jennifer walked into the antique shop, hoping to find a unique gift for her mother's birthday. She stumbled upon an old vase and decided it was perfect. That night, she dreamt of the vase shattering on the floor, revealing a hidden compartment with a strange key inside. When she woke up, she found the key in her hand. Jennifer went back to the antique shop to ask about the vase, but the owner had no memory of selling it. Instead, he gave her a map leading to a hidden treasure. As she followed the map, she encountered a strange man who offered her a deal – the treasure in exchange for a mysterious potion. Jennifer agreed and drank the potion, which transported her to a parallel universe. In this new world, she discovered that her father was alive and well, but she never existed in that reality. Jennifer had to choose between staying in this new world or returning to her own. She chose to go back, but the potion had a twist – she was sent back in time to the day she first found the vase. Now, with the knowledge of what was to come, Jennifer had the choice once again to return to her old life or stay and start anew. She decided to stay and as she explored this new timeline, she found that her actions had unforeseen consequences, both good and bad. Jennifer eventually found herself back in the antique shop, but this time, the owner remembered selling her the vase. He revealed that it was a magical object that granted wishes. Jennifer realized that her entire adventure was the result of her wish for a unique gift for her mother's birthday. Jennifer wished for everything to go back to normal. The vase shattered on the floor, just as she had dreamt, and she woke up in her own bed. She thought it was all just a dream, but when she went to her mother's birthday party, she found the exact same vase as the one in her dream, unbroken and sitting on the mantel.

That was a long winded story, but remember the negative that can come from what we think we want, every path carries bad and good

Surviving a World overturned by an AI EMP assault?

Strictly just some common sense, don't sue me if it happens and you forget to put your phone in a Faraday cage or drop it.

Securing Basic Needs: Water: Identify nearby water sources, such as rivers, lakes, or underground aquifers. Purify water before consumption using methods like boiling, filtration, or chemical disinfection.

Food: Prioritize non-perishable food items like canned goods, dry fruits, and energy bars. Forage for edible plants, berries, and insects while adhering to safety guidelines and avoiding potentially harmful species.

Maintaining Shelter: Find or construct a secure shelter to protect against environmental elements and AI surveillance. Utilize natural resources like caves, fallen trees, or makeshift structures using available materials. Minimize exposure to AI-controlled areas, focusing on remote locations or blending into abandoned urban areas with caution.

Navigating in a Disconnected World: Orient yourself using traditional navigation methods like compasses, maps, and celestial observations. Familiarize yourself with local landmarks and natural formations to aid navigation. Establish basic communication with trusted individuals using non-electronic means like whistles, signal fires, or improvised signaling devices.

Surviving AI Encounters: Stay vigilant and avoid contact with AI-controlled drones or surveillance systems. Learn to identify AI patterns and establish camouflage techniques to remain undetected. Develop a thorough understanding of AI behavior and adapt accordingly. Be prepared to change routes, hide, or seek alternate paths when necessary.

Coping with EMP Effects: Accept the loss of technological devices and adapt to a technology-free environment. Embrace traditional skills and manual tools for daily tasks. Seek natural sources of light, such as solar-powered lanterns or candles, and conserve resources to prolong their usage. Protect essential equipment and electronics in Faraday cages or shielding materials to shield them from further EMP damage.

Building Community: Establish connections and support networks with like-minded individuals who share your survival goals. Exchange knowledge, skills, and resources within the community to enhance collective resilience. Foster a sense of camaraderie and cooperation, working together to overcome challenges and rebuild a sustainable future.

In a pinch several layers of chicken wire or fine as possible conductive metal mesh sheets as possible, build a box all seems sealed, solid metals will work as well, but as long as the mesh is tighter then the overall height of the wave it should still provide some potential protections.

Squirrel Christmas
(Some are shunned)

In a village of squirrels
Deep within the woods
A chilling tradition
Shrouded in belief
With winter's arrival, a cruel rite takes place
When one squirrel faces exile
A haunting disgrace
Bound by ancient customs, they gather 'neath the trees
Whispering anxiously, on trembling knees
The Lottery commences, an ominous affair
As destiny's hand selects one squirrel in despair
The chosen squirrel, marked by fate's cruel hand
Bears the weight of the village, a forsaken stand
Banished from their home, cast into the unknown
Left to face the harsh winter, all alone
The villagers, with heavy hearts, turn a blind eye
Silencing their conscience, as traditions dictate
For fear and conformity weave a powerful spell
Binding them to the cycle, too deep to dispel
The youth, with hopeful eyes, question this decree
Yearning for change, a chance to break free
But the weight of tradition, a formidable force
Leaves their dreams shattered, their voices hoarse
And so, the Squirrel Lottery persists in its reign
A haunting reminder of a village's pain
Yet somewhere in the shadows, a spark may ignite
A glimmer of rebellion, a fight for what's right
For tradition's grip may falter, cracks start to show
As the seeds of dissent in young hearts grow
And one day, perhaps, the cycle will be undone
When the courage to challenge is kindled in someone
In this squirrel village, bound by tradition's hold
Dark secrets lie hidden, stories left untold
A cautionary tale of conformity's might
Where the price of tradition
Overshadows what's right

Though I do not wholly embrace all of the school of Stoicism I do look upon Marcus Aurelius in moments that I need some thought guidance, or to handle a situation. It became one of the base foundations along with Art of War at a young age to help me develop my masking skills to blend in with those around me. It humbled me and helped to shape my always smiling persona, it isn't always the healthiest mentally but at times survival is king.

The Red Balloon

Once upon a time, there was a red balloon. It was a bright and cheerful balloon, with a big smiley face on it. It lived in a big city where it would be bought by a little girl named Lily. She was a shy girl who often felt alone and unimportant. But when she held the red balloon, it made her feel happy and like she had a friend. Lily and the balloon went on many adventures together, exploring the city and having fun. But as time passed, Lily's life became harder. She struggled with anxiety and depression, and the red balloon became her only source of comfort. One day, while walking through the park, the balloon slipped out of Lily's hand and floated away. She felt devastated and alone, like she had lost her only friend. But as she sat on a bench and cried, she looked up and saw the balloon in the sky. It was flying higher and higher, going on an adventure of its own. And Lily realized that just like the balloon, she too could rise above her troubles and soar high. She didn't need the balloon to be happy, she could find happiness within herself. From that day on, Lily started taking care of herself. She went to therapy, talked to friends and family, and practiced self-care. She learned that she was important and worthy of love and happiness, and the red balloon became a symbol of her strength and resilience. The balloon eventually floated back down to Lily, but this time, she wasn't afraid to let it go. She knew that she could hold onto the memories of their adventures, but it was time to let the balloon fly free and take on new adventures of its own. And as the balloon floated away, Lily smiled and knew that no matter where it went, it would always hold a special place in her heart.

i prefer stuffies but to each their own.

LAUGH BREAK

Why did the tomato turn red? Because it saw the salad dressing!

What's the difference between a poorly dressed man on a trampoline and a well-dressed man on a trampoline? Attire.

What do you call a fake noodle? An imposta.

Why was the math book sad? Because it had too many problems.

What did the janitor say when he jumped out of the closet? "Supplies!"

Why can't you hear a pterodactyl go to the bathroom? Because the P is silent.

Why don't oysters share their pearls? Because they're shellfish.
I'm trying to organize a hide and seek tournament, but good players are hard to find.

Why did the coffee file a police report? It got mugged.

Why did the mathematician break up with his girlfriend? Because he realized that he could never truly divide his attention between her and his work, and that his obsession with numbers and equations had left him emotionally numb and incapable of forming meaningful connections with others. As he struggled to come to terms with this realization, he pushed her away and retreated further into his work, leaving behind a trail of broken relationships and shattered hearts. Eventually, he died alone, surrounded by his equations and the cold, unfeeling world of numbers that he had devoted his life to. LOL

broken perfects

In a world where
Everything was perfect,
The skies were always blue,
The sun always shone, and the
People always smiled. But there was
No passion, no struggle, and no real emotion.
Over time, the people grew numb and disconnected
From each other. Then, a stranger appeared with a somber
Face, speaking of a world beyond their own, full of pain and suf-
fering. He led them to a door, and some bravely stepped through,
unleashing a torrent of emotions they had never experienced. They
felt love and joy, but also pain and heartbreak. Initially, the people
recoiled in fear from these new sensations, but they soon realized
that they could only truly appreciate the good things in life by
Facing the bad. They learned that pain and suffering were a
Necessary part of being alive. As they integrated these
Lessons, the once-perfect world became richer and
More fulfilling than ever before. The stranger who
Showed them the way disappeared, but his legacy
Remained. The people had learned that life was
Not about avoiding pain and suffering, but
About embracing it as part of the
Human experience.

Sometimes numb is truly numb, and until you
know you can't. But when you do... I'm sorry

Haiku thoughts

Perfect world, hollow,
Yearning for something more,
Pain awaits beyond.

Faces twisted in
Tears and laughter, joy and pain,
World of emotion.

Life's dichotomy,
Pleasure cannot exist sans
Pain's duality.

The road less traveled
Leads to greater understanding,
Through trials and tears.

Embrace the darkness,
Find meaning in life's struggles,
Let pain be your guide.

In the depths of pain,
Light can be found shining bright,
Hope springs eternal.

In a perfect world, Emotionless and dull, Is it better to feel pain,
Or never feel at all?

Rainbow Days Dealership

A rainbow unicorn, prancing through the city. Cars honk and people stare as the unicorn passes by. The unicorn enters a car dealership, its hooves clicking against the linoleum floors. It looks around at the shiny cars on display and the serious-looking salespeople in suits. As the unicorn approaches the parts department, it sees a bald troll at the counter. The troll sneers and grumbles, "What do you want here, rainbow unicorn? This is a car dealership, not a fantasy land. We don't have any parts for your kind here."The unicorn, taken aback, tries to reason with the troll. "But I need a part for my rainbow horn. It's broken and I can't fix it without a new part."The troll just scoffs and turns away, leaving the unicorn frustrated and alone in the waiting room. The unicorn sits down in a chair, its long tail swishing back and forth. It tries to make small talk with the other customers, but no one seems interested in talking to a unicorn. Suddenly, the door bursts open and in walks a pickle. The pickle is wearing a top hat and carrying a cane. Everyone in the waiting room stares in shock. The pickle walks up to the unicorn and says, "Excuse me, sir, but do you know what the difference is between a pickle and a unicorn?" The unicorn, intrigued, shakes its head no. The pickle leans in and whispers, "Nothing. We're both just a little bit sour." Everyone in the waiting room erupts in laughter. Even the troll can't help but chuckle at the ridiculous sight of a pickle in a top hat. The unicorn realizes that maybe it doesn't need to belong in a car dealership to be happy. Maybe it's okay to be a little different. And with that realization, the unicorn's broken horn magically repairs itself, and it gallops out of the dealership, ready to take on the world. And the trolls hair magically grew back.

To bad you don't believe in magic Abe

mental warfare

In the dark recesses of the mind,
Where shadows lurk and fears entwine,
A battle rages day and night, As the soul struggles
To find the light. Voices whisper, taunting and cruel,
Tempting the heart to play the fool, Echoes of pain
And shattered dreams, Teeming with despair,
Or so it seems. But there is hope amidst
The fray, A spark of light to lead the
Way, A glimmer of truth, a guiding
Star, To help the wounded heart
Go far. Through the pain and
Endless strife, We learn
To navigate this life,
To rise above
The darkest hour,
And tap into our inner power.
For in the depths of mental pain,
We find the strength to rise again,
To face the darkness with a will, And let
Our inner light shine still. So take heart,
Weary traveler, Though the road be
Dark and treacherous, For in the end,
The battle won, You'll emerge
Into the rising sun.

*Just reach for the energy, when you cant seem to move, just picture yourself moving,
constantly pushing, constantly evolving, when you "cant" I tend to find you can.*

FURYCRAWL BOARD

Prepare for an adrenaline-fueled adventure like no other with the FuryCrawl, a colossal skateboard inspired by the resilience of the mighty centipede. This awe-inspiring beast is engineered to conquer the chaotic post-apocalyptic world, leaving a trail of awe and envy in its wake. Unleash Unparalleled Dominance: The FuryCrawl harnesses an unstoppable 16-wheel centipede configuration, defying gravity as it effortlessly maneuvers through the harshest terrains. Strap on the innovative MagneticGrip boots, instantly engaging with the built-in gyro stabilization system, ensuring unwavering control even on the most treacherous slopes. Embrace the Unexpected: Enhance your FuryCrawl experience with an array of awe-inspiring add-ons. Channel your inner firestarter with the PyroBlast flamethrower attachment, obliterating obstacles and leaving adversaries in awe of your ferocity. Scale towering structures with the ClawStrike grappling hook, granting you the freedom to conquer any obstacle that dares to stand in your way. Unparalleled Power and Agility: Crafted with the finest materials, the FuryCrawl stands tall and proud. Its colossal 10-inch wheels, akin to the centipede's formidable legs, provide superior traction and stability. With its flexible frame design and internal hinge mechanism, this mechanical marvel effortlessly adapts to the rugged terrain, delivering an exhilarating and smooth ride. Welcome to the Wasteland Revolution: Embrace the spirit of rebellion and embark on a journey that defies the laws of nature. With the FuryCrawl as your trusted companion, you become an unstoppable force, leaving a trail of epic tales in your wake. Join the ranks of the fearless and conquer the desolate wasteland like never before. Note: The FuryCrawl's immense size and weight will leave bystanders in awe, as it dominates the landscape with unyielding power and presence. Brace yourself for the ultimate adventure, where chaos and excitement collide. Are you prepared to embark on an extraordinary journey with the FuryCrawl? Unleash your inner daredevil, seize the wasteland, and let the FuryCrawl become your vessel to newfound freedom!

So can I use the grappling hook and the flamethrowers at the same time? Kinda asking for a friend. Like imagine you are spinning on the way straight up the side of a bridge and just launching fire all around you on your rise... it's beautiful.

Siren Call of Sleep

sleep, sleep, my love, and do not fear,
the demons that haunt inside of here.
for when the night is at its darkest,
that's when your stars can shine the brightest.
close your eyes, my dear,
let your worries disappear,
deep inside your mind,
peace and calm you'll find.
quiet now, my child,
rest your head and close your eyes,
though your thoughts may roam,
you are safe here in your home,
your safe space where you can be alone.
sleep, sleep, my love, and do not fear,
the demons that haunt inside of here.
for when the night is at its darkest,
that's when your stars can shine the brightest.
in your dreams i guess you'll find
all the answers to your mind,
whispers from your soul
will help you apparently reach your goal.
sleep oh sweet sleep my love i aimlessly seek,
and do not fear the demons that you've created
here.
for when the night is at its darkest and your
life taste of nothing but tartness
that's when the stars shine the brightest, but
only
if you the strength to guide them.

close your eyes, my dear,
sleep away your pain and fear,
for when the dawn breaks new,
you'll find strength to see you through.

Oh so sleep is the magical answer? Well that explains a lot. I don't tend to do much of that.

ACROSTIC SUNSHINE

Delighted to be alive

Every moment a new chance

People all around me

Resting in the sunshine

Escaping from life's troubles

Savoring every breath

Simply enjoying the ride

Excited for what's to come

Dancing through each day

As we dance through life struggles may come
Even when we smile let us seek help and support
Please don't suffer alone, EVERY DAY is a NEW BEGINNING
Sing out for joy and love smile and embrace each moment

WANDERING MIND

In a world of thoughts, a mind does wander,
                    Seeking solace from the mental thunder.
A symphony of chaos, thoughts collide,
                    A restless sea where tranquility hides.
But fear not, my friend, for within this storm,
                    There lies a refuge, a place to transform.
Through art and words, a portal emerges,
                    Where thoughts find shape and the mind converges.
A painter's brush, a poet's pen,
                    Unleash the magic, let creation begin.
In colors and verses, dreams take flight,
                    Transforming darkness into radiant light.
With each stroke, a universe unfurls,
                    A melody played, the soul's voice twirls.
The mind's torrential waves find their peace,
                    As creativity brings a sweet release.
So let your imagination soar and play,
                    For in creation, worries drift away.
Through art's embrace, find solace and rest,
                    And let your heart sing, feeling truly blessed.
In every stroke and every rhyme,
                    Discover the power to transcend time.
Embrace the muse that whispers in your ear,
                    And let your creations chase away all fear.
For in the realm of art, we find our grace,
                    A sanctuary where souls find their place.
So let the beauty of your creations be,
                    A balm for others, setting their spirits free.

If we never get lost, how could we ever begin to find ourselves? Most know where they are, not who they are. They see where they are in life and accept that as life, go for a walk and I don't mean physically.

flip book

In this flip book of
Life's grand design,
Pages flip with
Chaos intertwined.
Accept the world
In all its shades,
For within its twists,
True beauty pervades.
The chapters turn,
Emotions rise and fall,
Dark and whimsy dance,
Entwined in a ball.
Through highs and lows,
We learn and grow,
Embracing every color of the show.
The whimsical twists bring laughter's delight,
A sprinkle of magic in the darkest night.
But don't shy away from shadows that creep,
For they hold lessons
We're meant to keep. Acceptance,
The key to find inner peace,
Embracing imperfections,
Seeking release.
In the chaos,
We find strength to cope,
Navigating life's kaleidoscope.
So let us flip through each fleeting page,
Finding solace in this wild,
Wondrous stage.
Embrace the whimsy,
The dark and the bright,
For within this flip book, we truly ignite.

I enjoy thinking of the world, and life itself in more interest-
ing forms, almost creating well literally a flip book and take my
thoughts and issues and put them on the page before me, visual it
as if it was a book and try to imagine how it looks as an outsider.

Read me first!!!!!!!

Hello! So what kinda book do you have in your hand? What exactly will it say to you, what will it lead you to, and what will it evolve into? What at this point in the book I'm just as clueless as you are, maybe less so even. It's not like I started it with a plan or anything specific in mind, I have tried that, I have books upon books of planned stories. What this will be isn't that, poems are nice, short stories, and random thoughts along the way. I'm not going to be your one trick pony, maybe you laugh, maybe you cry, and maybe just maybe you fall in love.... Don't know why you would just seems like an emotion that went with that whole thing. What is this really? The mental ramblings that keep coming forth from this beautiful spectral dark rainbow that I call my sideways flipped autistic mind, oh what? Yeah squirrel moments bound to come. But hell I'm ready to see where this goes, like those bird soup for the feels books except more like Ramen for the 4th dimensional self. Maybe spicy ramen.... throw some pork in that. Oh right, get to reading.

**This world will be the death of me.
I mean no shit right? Isn't that the point?**

After this you can flip to any page.

If that's the point, then why do so many of us spend our lives trying to escape it? Trying to find meaning in something greater than ourselves? Maybe it's because deep down, we all know that this world is a beautiful, chaotic, and ultimately meaningless place. But that doesn't mean we can't find joy and purpose in the moments we have. So read on, dear reader, and see what this book has to offer. Maybe you'll find something worth holding on to. Or maybe you'll just be reminded that we're all just along for the ride.

That's it, that's all I got. Well actually what you are about to read is just the tip the iceberg, let's keep this random pages of madness going, pass me around, between classes you can share me, you don't even need a bookmark just go to any page and flip as you please, we all need random and some of us can jump so far in-between. Take a breath, take a break, and read, but don't flip through the pages, I'm short yes, and seemingly unrelated, but every one of them can mean something deeper if you take a minute and think of them, some books need breathes in between pages, let something soak before you forget it, when the world gets dark one random thought might save your head in one dark hole. I'm random so welcome to my world. :)

"But hey, isn't that the beauty of life? We get to experience all the ups and downs, the highs and lows, the joys and sorrows. It's what makes us human, what makes us feel alive. So why not embrace it and make the most of the time we have?"

don't ask why

All around us,
Chaos and mess,
But don't let
It bring
You
Distress.
Life can
Be hard, that's
No lie, But keep
Your chin up, don't
Ask why. The world's not
Perfect, that's for sure, But don't
Let it be your only lure. There's beauty
In the darkness too, A different light that
Shines for you. Embrace the sadness, feel the
Pain, But don't let it consume your brain. You're
Stronger than you know, my friend, Your journey's
Not yet at its end. So when the storm clouds start to
gather, And life feels like an endless blather, Remember
that the sun will shine, And brighter days will soon
Be thine. So take my hand and we'll stand tall,
Together we can conquer all. With hope and
Love and grit and grace, We'll find
Our way to a brighter place.

When I say "don't ask why" it is to drive the idea that it
can't really solve much normally, yes motive is important but
don't let the confusion of the why cloud your ability to act.

Haiku thoughts

Embrace the chaos,
Breathe in life's unpredictable,
Find peace in the storm.

Life's twists and turns,
A never-ending journey,
Take the path with grace.

The sun sets each day,
Yet the dawn always arrives,
New beginnings bloom.

Winter's cold embrace,
Melts into spring's warm embrace,
Nature's constant dance.

Even in darkness,
Stars shine in the endless night,
Hope amidst the void.

Rain falls from above,
A cleansing of the spirit,
Nature's therapy.

Accepting the things we cannot change and changing the things that we can. This is an important lesson in life, it helps us separate our thoughts with the things that are needed now and the things we can ponder on later. And helps to give focus to a scatter brain.

Surviving an Island full of Sea Scorpions?

Strictly just some common sense, don't sue me if it happens and you make the perfect spear and after crafting it take it to show it off and trip and fall on it.

Maintain Distance: Sea scorpions may be aggressive if provoked or threatened. Keep a safe distance from their nesting grounds or any areas where they are known to inhabit. Avoid sudden movements that could attract their attention and incite an attack.

Identify Safe Zones: Scout the island's terrain for natural formations or structures that offer protection against sea scorpions. Caves, rock formations, or sturdy shelters can serve as refuge, providing a barrier between you and the dangerous creatures.

Create Barriers: If you're unable to find a suitable shelter, construct a barrier using available materials. Use rocks, logs, or any other large objects to create a physical barrier that prevents the sea scorpions from reaching you. Be mindful of potential entry points and fortify them to minimize the risk of infiltration.

Protective Clothing: Wear thick, protective clothing that covers your body, including long sleeves, pants, and closed-toe shoes. This will reduce the likelihood of sea scorpions' stingers penetrating your skin. Consider using thick gloves or arm guards for added protection.

Avoid Bright Colors: Sea scorpions are attracted to bright colors, considering them potential prey. Wear clothing in earth tones or camouflage patterns to blend in with the surroundings and minimize the chances of drawing their attention.

Stay Still in Water: Sea scorpions are primarily aquatic creatures. If you find yourself in the water with them nearby, remain as still as possible. Thrashing or making sudden movements can attract their attention and trigger an attack. Slowly back away from their vicinity while maintaining calm.

Craft Weapons: If you must defend yourself, craft simple weapons using materials from the island. Sharpened sticks, spears, or makeshift slingshots can provide a means of deterrence or distraction. Aim for their sensory organs or vulnerable spots to maximize the effectiveness of your strikes.

Seek Higher Ground: Sea scorpions may have limited mobility on land. If the island offers elevated terrain, seek higher ground to increase your safety. Climb trees, cliffs, or any elevated structures where sea scorpions would struggle to reach you.

Call for Help: If there's a chance of rescue, use any available means to signal for assistance. Build a signal fire, use a signaling mirror or whistle, or create visible markings on the beach to attract attention from passing boats or aircraft.

Stay Calm and Observant: Panicking in the presence of sea scorpions can cloud your judgment and increase the risk of making hasty, ill-advised decisions. Stay calm, observe their behavior from a safe distance, and use your knowledge of their patterns to plan your next move strategically.

I remember a time that sea scorpions weren't my worst fear, but you know there's worse fears. Heights, being upside down, walrus, flaming tennis balls, this one dragon named Gimbo, actually scratch all this, I'll delete it later. Sea scorpions still win.. Almost forgot about peanut butter sticking to the roof of my mouth.

Puzzle Box

In a dimly lit room, shrouded in mystery's embrace,a man grappled with a puzzling case. The puzzle box taunted him, its enigma unfurled, but every attempt was thwarted, his progress unfurled. With each grasp, a strange occurrence inter-vened,
An eerie presence that left him disconcerted and keen. The room's atmosphere turned icy and cold,as if unseen forces delighted in his stronghold. Undeterred, he persisted, driven by obsession,haunted by the puzzle's allure, an enigmatic possession.

Yet, the room played tricks, shadows danced on the wall,leaving him on edge, his sanity on the brink of a fall. But he pressed on, determined to unlock its secret,unaware of the darkness lurking, growing discreet. Whispers echoed, chilling his spine, as he delved deeper into the puzzle's confine. The room, an accomplice to his descent,an orchestration of chaos, twisted and bent. Objects defied gravity, defying the laws, while the man unraveled, lost in its claws.

In his final attempt, desperation consumed his soul, but laughter echoed, as if from a demonic troll. The room plunged into darkness, a chilling void, revealing the puzzle's insidious ploy. Inside the box, a snapshot picture reflection of him trying to solve the puzzle box, a cruel mockery, an impossible trap that would severe his reality. The room laughed, his fate sealed in despair,forever trapped, a puppet in the puzzle's snare. Within those walls, his efforts all in vain, he realized some mysteries brought only pain. The puzzle box, a portal to a realm untold, a sinister riddle that left his sanity on hold. The laughter lingered, a haunting refrain, as he descended into madness, forever detained. A prisoner of his own insatiable curiosity,
Trapped in the depths of a twisted reality.

In that room, shadows danced with delight,the man's existence swallowed by eternal night. This a tale of a mind consumed, by the puzzles that ensnare, leaving souls entombed.

Sometimes the urge to know something is so strong that our own abilities and weaknesses seem to disappear, everything we know, everything we hold close seems to be so far away, and the rest of the world goes black, it ends with only the item in question and the answer, nothing else matters, food loses all meaning, time seems to melt to nothingness, and space itself almost breathes in a bubble around you, and everything else is a distant echo. Hyper focus has taken control.

PERIODIC TABLE OF THE ELEMENTS

1A	2A	3B	4B	5B	6B	7B	8B	8B	8B	1B	2B	3A	4A	5A	6A	7A	8A
1 H 1.008																	2 He 4.003
3 Li 6.939	4 Be 9.0122											5 B 10.811	6 C 12.011	7 N 14.007	8 O 15.999	9 F 18.998	10 Ne 20.183
11 Na 22.99	12 Mg 24.312											13 Al 26.982	14 Si 28.086	15 P 30.974	16 S 32.064	17 Cl 35.453	18 Ar 39.948
19 K 39.102	20 Ca 40.08	21 Sc 44.956	22 Ti 47.9	23 V 50.942	24 Cr 51.996	25 Mn 54.938	26 Fe 55.847	27 Co 58.933	28 Ni 58.71	29 Cu 63.546	30 Zn 65.37	31 Ga 69.72	32 Ge 72.59	33 As 74.922	34 Se 78.96	35 Br 79.904	36 Kr 83.8
37 Rb 85.47	38 Sr 87.62	39 Y 88.905	40 Zr 91.22	41 Nb 92.906	42 Mo 95.94	43 Tc [97]	44 Ru 101.07	45 Rh 102.91	46 Pd 106.4	47 Ag 107.87	48 Cd 112.4	49 In 114.82	50 Sn 118.69	51 Sb 121.75	52 Te 127.6	53 I 126.9	54 Xe 131.3
55 Cs 132.91	56 Ba 137.34	57* La 138.91	72 Hf 178.49	73 Ta 180.95	74 W 183.85	75 Re 186.2	76 Os 190.2	77 Ir 192.2	78 Pt 195.09	79 Au 196.97	80 Hg 200.59	81 Tl 204.37	82 Pb 207.19	83 Bi 208.98	84 Po 210	85 At 210	86 Rn 222
87 Fr 215	88 Ra 226.03	89** Ac 227.03	104 Rt [261]	105 Db [262]	106 Sg [266]	107 Bh [264]	108 Hs [269]	109 Mt [268]	110 [271]	111 [272]	112 [277]		114 [289]		116 [289]		

*Lanthanides	58 Ce 140.12	59 Pr 140.91	60 Nd 144.24	61 Pm 145	62 Sm 150.35	63 Eu 151.96	64 Gd 157.25	65 Tb 158.92	66 Dy 162.5	67 Ho 164.93	68 Er 167.26	69 Tm 168.93	70 Yb 173.04	71 Lu 174.97	
**Actinides	90 Th 232.04	91 Pa 231	92 U 238.03	93 Np 237.05	94 Pu 239.05	95 Am 241.06	96 Cm 244.06	97 Bk 249.08	98 Cf 252.08	99 Es 252.08	100 Fm 257.1	101 Md 258.1	102 No 259.1	103 Lr 262.11	

Gaseous at room temperature
Liquid at room temperature
Gallium melts at 29.78 deg. C.
Synthetic elements
All other elements are solid at room temperature

LETTER TO SELF

Dear Past Self,

As a cosmic explorer, I pen this letter to guide you through the vastness of life. Embrace the infinite possibilities that lie before you. Be fearless in the face of uncertainty, for within the unknown lies extraordinary growth. Embrace both triumphs and failures, for they are the markers of your journey. Nurture your dreams with unwavering belief and unwavering dedication. Let them guide you like the stars in the night sky, illuminating your path. And when doubts arise, find solace within your own being, for you possess immense strength and resilience. Along this cosmic voyage, seek kindred spirits who share your vision and ignite your soul. Together, form constellations of friendship, shining brightly amidst the darkness. Cherish these connections, for they will provide comfort and inspiration in times of need. Remember, dear self, that the universe is a tapestry of wonders waiting to be discovered. Embrace the mysteries that unfold before you, and let your curiosity be your guiding star. The cosmos beckons you with open arms, inviting you to embark on extraordinary adventures. With boundless love and cosmic energy,

Your Future Self

I find these very helpful and therapeutic to write and read, because even if you aren't where you want to be you can think back at where you have been and share experiences with that version of yourself. Things to remember and lessons learned.

Surviving an Encounter with a Time Vortex?
Strictly just some common sense, don't sue me if it happens and you accidentally stop your parents meeting.

Maintain Calm: Stay composed and do not panic when confronted with the unknown.

Observe Surroundings: Take note of any unusual phenomena or distortions in the environment. Look for recognizable landmarks or objects that may provide clues about your location in time.

Preserve Personal Safety: Prioritize your safety and well-being at all times. Stay away from hazardous areas or potential dangers caused by temporal anomalies.

Preserve Mental Stability: Coping with time displacement can be disorienting and emotionally challenging. Focus on maintaining a clear and stable mindset to make rational decisions.

Gather Information: Try to gather information about the time period you find yourself in. Observe clothing styles, architecture, language, and cultural cues to determine the era.

Blend In: Dress appropriately to blend in with the time period.
Avoid drawing unnecessary attention to yourself to prevent disruption of the timeline.

Seek Local Assistance: Approach local authorities or individuals who may be able to assist you. Exercise caution in revealing details about your origin or time travel experience.

Adapt to Resources: Adjust to the available resources and technology of the time period. Learn basic survival skills that may be necessary for that era, such as foraging or fire-making.

Maintain Hope: Stay positive and resilient despite the challenges of being displaced in time. Keep a focus on finding a way back to your original timeline, if desired.

Document Your Experience: Keep a record of your experiences, observations, and any information that may assist you in future attempts to return to your own time.

I wonder if we would just kinda phase out, cease to exist, or maybe because we don't exist no one keeps our parents from meeting and so they actually do meet, and we come back into existence just to repeat the cycle endlessly.. So maybe don't do anything like that, also don't hit on your great grand parents in their time line. It's weird.

Heart's Song

In a world of vibrant hues, where colors danced and twirled
There lived a boy in hidden pain, his spirit tightly furled
Cloaked in hoodies, a shield to hide his scars
He walked through life, unnoticed, beneath the shimmering stars
His sleeves cascaded, a veil for secret strife
Yet his heart yearned for freedom, to embrace his hidden life
Silent, he listened to the voices all around
Never uttering a no, his voice forever bound
But deep within his soul, a melody longed to be sung
A song of truth and courage, from a place so deeply wrung
And one day, with trembling lips, he dared to let it out
But the notes stumbled and faltered, his voice filled with doubt
Rainbow tears poured forth, each droplet like a prism's glow
A symphony of emotions, his heart's overflow
They streamed down his face, painting the world anew
As his tears told a story only colors could construe
The world, enchanted by this spectacle so rare
Listened intently to the silent cries in the air
And as the boy wept, a harmony arose
A chorus of humming, a melody that chose
From every corner of existence, voices joined in tune
A resounding hum that echoed under the moon
The boy, astounded, witnessed his tears transform
Into a symphony of colors, his pain now a platform
No longer confined by the chains of silent despair
He found solace in his song, an embrace beyond compare
With each note he mustered, his voice grew bold and free
A testament to his spirit, a testament to be
For in the realm of colors, he discovered his own worth
His scars a tapestry of strength, a testament to rebirth
And as his voice soared, embracing the vast unknown
He found his true essence, a vibrant light brightly shown

To learn from this boy, his journey bittersweet
To embrace our own uniqueness, our true selves to greet
For in the kaleidoscope of life, we all have our own song
Let it echo through the universe, and forever sing along

TEMPERED LOVE

Once
Upon a time,
A little girl, Fought
Through the flames
That consumed
Her world,
Her father's
Anger, burning
Bright Against her
Crib, a tragic sight As
She grew, she battled on
Against the darkness, and all
That's wrong But the world can
Be a cruel place And she often fell,
Without a trace, She struggled with
Herself and others, In a world filled with
Confusion and blunders, But through the
Trials, she
Persevered
And with
Each step,
She overcame
Her
Fears,
And in time, she built a
Family of her own, A loving group, with
Seeds of hope sown, Her past may have been a raging fire,
But she emerged stronger, rising ever higher, Through the
trials and the tests of life, She learned to stand tall, and
face the strife, For though the world may be a cruel place,
There is always hope, and a chance
To embrace, And so she lived, with heart
And soul, And taught her children, to be
Bold, For though the journey may be
Long, With love and courage,
We all belong.

Every story has a backup story remember that, every character whether the hero or the villain or something in-between. Character is built, it doesn't justify but it does teach. - SRV

fill in the blank you

In a walnut factory, a pig did dwell
Lost in the maze, a peculiar spell
Through rows of nuts, it wandered astray
Seeking an escape, day after day
In search of freedom, it climbed up high
Upon a bull, mechanical and spry
With each twist and turn, it aimed for the sky
Determined to reach the window nearby
But fate had a twist, as the dragon soared
Breaking the ceiling, its fiery roar
The pig was startled, its mission disrupted
As the dragon's flames, the scene erupted
And in that moment, the tale took a turn

A shift in the narrative, we must discern
Apologies for the abrupt change in flow
The previous tale's end, for now, is unknown
Yet let us cherish the pig's brave quest
To conquer challenges and do its best
Though the story may seem incomplete
Imagination's journey remains a treat

So I guess the end of this one is up to you, are you in a good mood
or a bad mood? Cooked bacon or maybe magical ice that freezes
the dragon's flames, or maybe a walnut gets lodged in something
and catapults into the dragon's eye and distracts it. Just use your
imagination dang it, I can't finish them all.

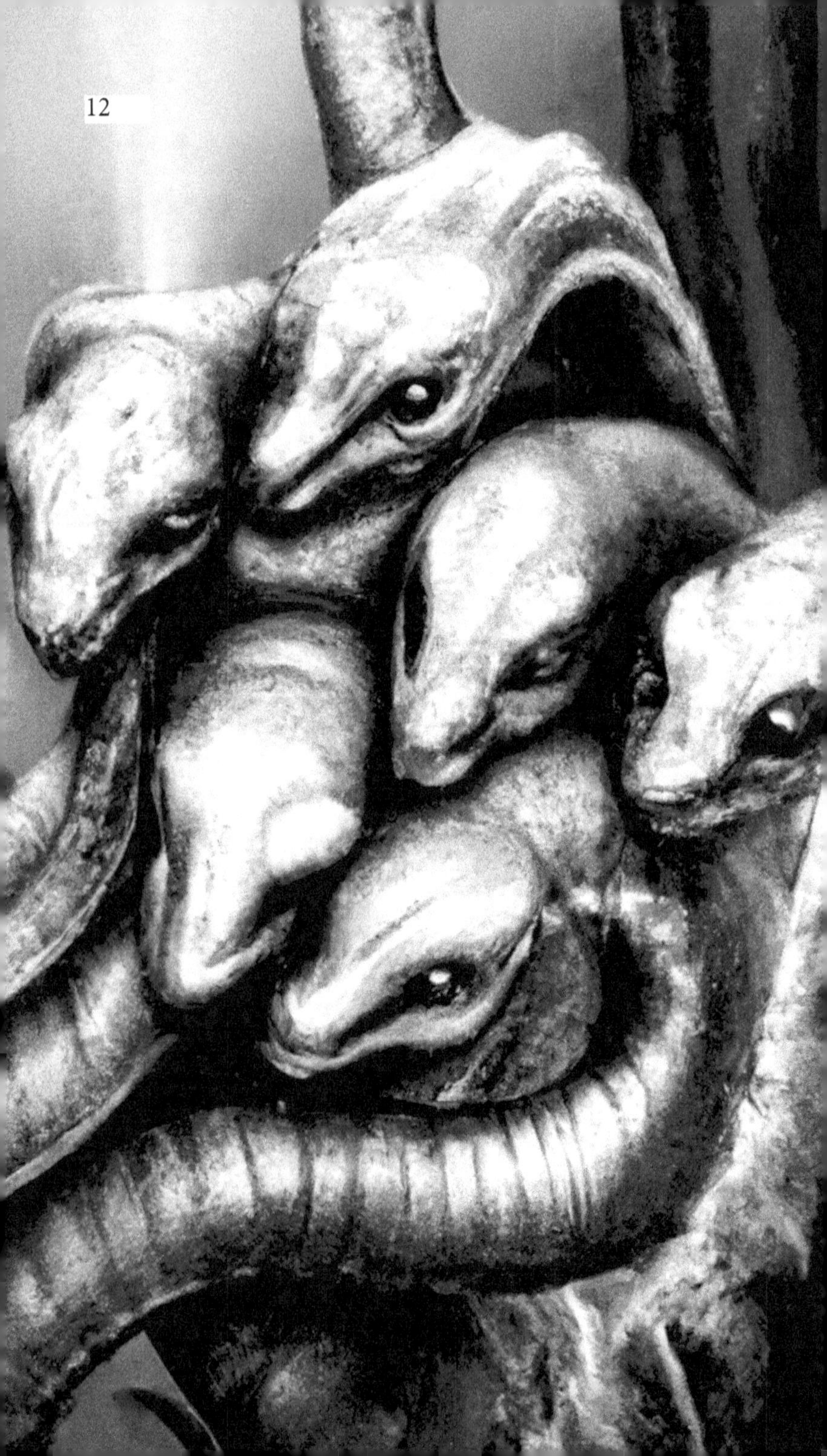

Rainbow Wall

In a
World of
Color a rainbow
Gleams, Painting the
Sky with vibrant dreams
Arching high, its hues so bright
A dazzling spectacle, a wondrous sight
But as the storm brews, winds start to
Blow, The rainbow transforms, its purpose
To show, With a shimmering grace, it takes a
Stand, Turning into a wall of light, so grand, a
Humble home, made of mud and love, Stands in the
Tornado's path, unwavering and tough, as the swirling
Winds threaten to destroy, The rainbow's light shields
Radiating joy, brick by brick, the wall is built, defending
The home with unwavering tilt, with colors still shining
Hope fills the air, protecting the cherished
Dwelling with care, amidst the chaos
The storm's mighty roar, the
Rainbow's light embraces
Forevermore
A beacon of strength
A guardian so bold, shielding the home
A story to be told
So remember this tale
When troubles arise
That even a rainbow can wear a disguise
In times of danger
Love will prevail
Building walls of light
That never fail

Sometimes we can be whatever we need to be, it isn't always what is in our nature,
But change is very important, it is also very difficult, most of us don't really want to change
But we learn to embrace it as we go, it's the only way at times to survive
Be a rainbow, be anything and everything, be yourself and allow your colours to shine.

UNIVERSAL LAWS

THE LAW OF BALANCE
HARMONY IN ALL ASPECTS
PEACE WITHIN ONESELF.

THE LAW OF FOCUS
THE MIND CONTROLS THE BODY
CONCENTRATE TO GROW.

THE LAW OF KARMA
INTENTIONS DETERMINE FATE
GOOD DEEDS BEAR FRUIT SOON.

THE LAW OF NATURE
CHANGE IS THE ONLY CONSTANT
EVOLVE ADAPT THRIVE.

THE LAW OF RHYTHM
LIFE FLOWS IN UPS AND DOWNS
ENDURE PERSEVERE.

THE LAW OF UNITY
CONNECTEDNESS OF ALL THINGS
ONE IN DIVERSITY.

Balance is so hard of a concept, and inner peace or outer peace? Kinda looks like I typed otter peace, but I don't really know if they have much war... sooooooo.... Find inner focus or dancing or something.. Distracted by otter war fantasy..

shine and play

Once upon
A time in a world of wonder,
Lived a young girl who felt like a thunder. She loved to
Dance and sing and play, But the world told her to stay away.
"You're too loud," they said with a frown, "Be quiet and small,
Don't make a sound." So she hid herself away, Afraid to be
Herself and play. But one day a wise old owl, Came to her
With a howl, "Be yourself, don't hide away, Let your
Colours shine and play." So the young girl took a
Stand,
And danced and sang
Across the land.
Her colors shining
Bright,
Like a rainbow
In the sky at night.
And though some still
Told her to be quiet,
She knew that being
Herself was her true riot.
So she danced and
Sang and played,
And never let the world make her afraid.

Not gonna lie here, I was trying to shape this like a flower, fun fact all flower shapes have to exist somewhere in this universe right? So I drew a flower. Fact. Be yourself, it's important, this world will try to break you, just break back.

LAST WILL AND TESTAMENT

Old man Johnson
Had finally passed away and his lawyer
Was reading his last will and testament to the family.
"To my eldest son, John, I leave my house and my car," the lawyer said.
Then he continued, "To my youngest son, Peter, I leave my bike and my laptop."
"And to my daughter, Sarah, I leave my big-screen TV and my favorite couch," the lawyer
finished. The family was surprised,
Thinking the will would be much more substantial.
But then the lawyer
Pulled out a small envelope
And said, "And to all of you, I leave my most prized possession."
The family leaned in, wondering what it could be.
The lawyer opened the envelope
And pulled out a single sheet of paper.
He read aloud,
"To all of you, I leave my unpaid bills."

Does this count as a joke? We can't ever really expect anything in this life though, nothing is every promised to us beyond the moment and breath that we draw this very moment, find ourselves lucky if we find the same is true the next day.

CYBERFOOT

Gather 'round the fire, my friends,
For a tale that chills and sends shivers through your spine,
In the deep, dark woods, where legends abound, Lurks a creature
so fearsome, a terror so profound. They call it the Cyberfoot, a
monstrous sight. Half-machine, half-beast, a creature of the night,
With eyes glowing red and a mechanical growl, It hunts electronics,
ready to pounce and prowl even when your phone is on silence, Its
footsteps are heavy, like thunder on the ground, Leaving tracks that
bewilder, nowhere to be found, A retractable grappling hand, sharp
as a knife, Snatches unsuspecting prey, ending their life. In its metal
claws, a gleaming meat cleaver, A weapon of choice, a harbinger of
terror, The Cyberfoot roams through the trees,
A nightmare made real,
Causing hearts to freeze.
Those who dare cross its path, beware,
For it shows no mercy, no compassion, no care,
It hunts with precision, relentless and cold,
Leaving a trail of horror, stories yet untold.
So huddle close, my friends, by the campfire's light,
Keep your eyes open, vigilant through the night,
For Cyberfoot could be very close, just waiting for a ping,
To triangulate your final location.

So we all have to be thinking the same thing here right? Like who is making these
things and putting them in the wild? Yes crazy stories scary and blah blah blah, but
how is the reader suppose to make the leap that their was a government program
that created these creatures in the late 80's to hunt rogue pop stars until everybody
started carrying cellphones and well..bears.

WHERE WE BEGAN AGAIN

When you start to feel it coming it's almost to late
The gnawing and gnashing is around the corner and you can hear the approach
You run up to a house with a lit porch light and bang on the door
The creature begins to rustle the tall grass as you start kicking at the door
It opens and a little girl with big blue eyes and a yellow flower print dress is standing there
She tells you "This is my older Sister's house, she isn't in right now."
You explain the situation as she looks behind you at the grass that has since gone quiet
She looks you over once more "Everything is going to be okay outside, but inside is still an
option, come in if you want, just remember to shut the door on the way in."
The grass began to rustle again and you can see a hand trying to reach out of the bush
But it seemed to freeze in place before it made it into the yard
You step into the doorway and it seems as if the thing chasing you drops it's hands in
defeat. The girl speaks up "Sister insist on shutting the door, can't have ones moving about.
Proper manners of course, you shut the door and as the mechanism clicks into place and
sharp cracking sound. Had you really broken the door? Someone takes you in and....
All of a sudden a flash of light catches your attention and the little girl screams...
Had the creature gotten inside, had it followed you? The same familiar growl that you had
heard hours before, the first time you saw that weird creature with yellow eyes chasing
you, it had followed you this whole distance and you had rode your bike until you couldn't
clear the rocky path, and then you had ran, and ran and still it was right there. You could
now almost hear it, a mechanical growl grating against the outside of the window...
The outside of the window.."I can't ever seem to get it right, I try to stop me, and I can't,
I never listen, I scream that it's a trap and still I never listen, I tell myself that I will do
better and I still never get up enough strength to break the cycle, I always wind up inside,
please just remember, this is only the worst part, but we have tried, so many mes have
screamed until our throats bleed, until our nails tear from our fingers and our eyes have
Burst from every vessel, but still we continue, we fall into the trap."
The little girl screams again, and you turn and follow. The creature outside had confused
you, but you still had to see what was wrong with the girl. You can hear her again as you
turn into the hallway, "I told you if you stayed outside you would be safe, I'm so tired of
watching this." The mounted flamethrowers begin to singe the back of your legs as you
jump out of the way, no turning around you head forward, needles litter the floor points
facing up at weird angles, sheets of paper thinly line the walls which appear to be made of
glass, as you tear it away you see the maze before you, and begin to remember the lives
that stood behind you, time tends to turn in cycles, you can't escape this maze, you make it
three more hallways before you finally fall into a pit breaking your legs while the overhead
flamethrower finishes the job, you feel the split, and see a man, he looks like you, you
approach him and start screaming for him to turn around... he run towards the house.

Some say everything is a maze inside a maze inside a maze.. I say my head hurts

Tormented elves

It stands to reason that things exist beyond our recognition
Things that seem to be right on the edge of something more then
What we believe is possible. These creatures with yellow eyes
have been known for eons as Tormented Elves. It is a translation
error but we will get to that later. The tormented part isnt the
translation error though and I wish it was. Imagine if every
nerve
In your body was on set on fire at once, and then all of a sudden
you are fine. you approach the flame once again
Without knowing what is waiting. without knowing what could
happen. and then it does. it burns you again
And again. and again. and again
You forget. but the pain doesnt
The ether doesnt. it burns your very
Soul. the very core of your being. the creation
of this creature is no secret. they exist within loops of endless time
Created in cosmic jokes. special locations that can exist just slightly
beyond time. The Old Makers at times allow dark creations to
manifest within these areas and they choose at times to capture
innocent bystanders. and torment them with the only rule from
the Old Makers being the person must enter each time by their
own free will... If only the words of the dead carried outside the
trap. the true loss in translation here was of course the elves... it
was never elves. but anyone that knew well enough that it was
Tormented Selves choose to say very little about it..

The Old Makers Collection of Creatures, Created in very
Unique Ways. Put concentrated pain? We got you, and
next up maybe check out -28 for another Old Maker
Special.

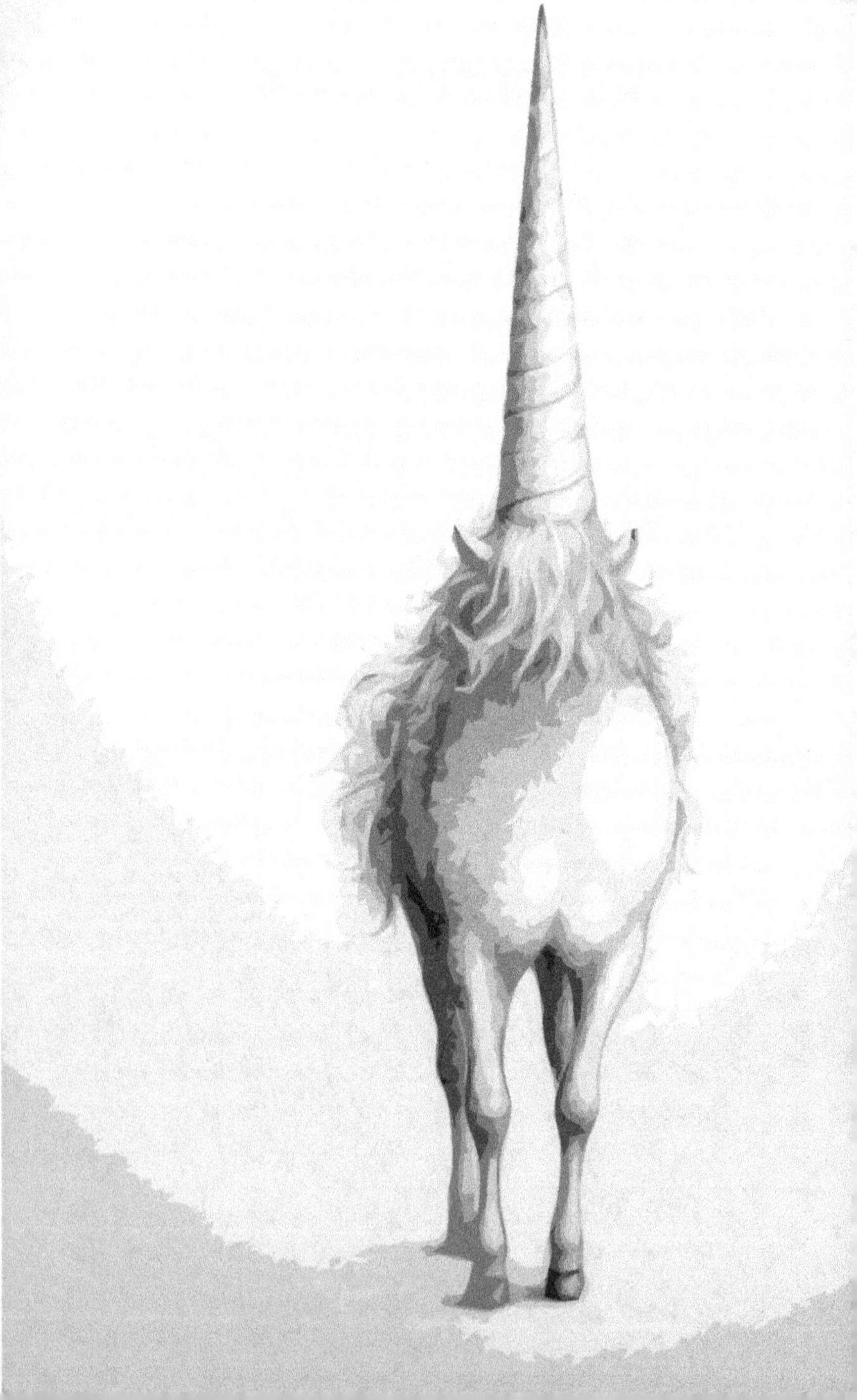

Cosmic Journeys

CELESTIAL DANCES, SOARS HIGH
STARDUST DREAMS
VAST SKY
OPAL HUES
SAPPHIRE EMBRACE
ASTRAL VOYAGE, TIME AND
SPACE, GOLDEN SPARKS, RUBY GLOW
COSMIC SYMPHONY, HEART'S ECHO
THREADS ENTWINED
FOREVER BOUND
VIBRANT REALM
COLORS PROFOUND
CELESTIAL PATHS
STARS ALIGN
TRANSCEND WORDS
SOULS INTERTWINE
FIRE OF COSMOS
DREAMS TAKE FLIGHT
EMBRACING WONDERS
INFINITE LIGHT
DUST REBORN, ART UNFOLDS
HEART'S VOYAGE
STORIES UNTOLD
GUIDED BY HEAVENS
REALMS FREE
EXPLORING COSMIC
TAPESTRY
ESSENCE OF STARS
SPIRIT'S QUEST
CANVAS AGLOW
DIVINE BEQUEST
GUIDED BY WONDERS
WANDERING FREE
THROUGH REALMS OF
COSMIC ECSTASY

A peace can be found on exploring something beyond physical. I mean honestly you might call me crazy, but have you ever tried? Have you ever put an honest effort into trying to explore your own mind, exploring yourself almost as if it was a road trip and you are a passenger in your own life, try to weigh and measure things through this perspective, almost out of body and into mind.

 # Surviving in a Jungle After a Plane Crash?
Strictly just some common sense, don't sue me if it happens and you have to eat your own leg.

After the Crash: Assess yourself for injuries. Attend to any immediate life-threatening conditions and provide first aid to others if possible. Evacuate the aircraft promptly and move away from it to a safe distance. Once you're a safe distance away, take a headcount to ensure all survivors are accounted for.

Stay Positive and Calm: Maintain a positive mindset and stay focused on survival.
Take deep breaths and manage stress to conserve energy and make rational decisions.

Find or Build Shelter: Seek natural shelters like caves or overhanging cliffs. Construct a shelter using available materials like branches, leaves, and debris.

Locate Water Sources: Look for nearby streams, rivers, or pools of water. Collect rainwater using natural catchment methods or create a solar still.

Gather Food: Identify edible plants, fruits, and nuts in the jungle. Learn basic trapping techniques to catch small game or fish.

Fire Starting: Collect dry wood, leaves, and tinder for fire. Use primitive fire-starting methods like a fire plow or bow drill.

Navigation and Signaling: Learn to navigate using the sun, stars, and natural landmarks. Use reflective materials or mirrors to create signaling devices for attracting attention.

Wildlife and Hazards: Be cautious of poisonous plants and dangerous animals. Protect yourself from insect bites and create protective clothing.

Mental Strength and Rescue Efforts: Stay hopeful and maintain a routine to keep your spirits up. Create visible signals, such as large SOS signs or markers, to attract potential rescuers.

Remember, these are general guidelines, and specific survival techniques and priorities may vary depending on the location, climate, and resources available in the jungle. It's crucial to prepare by acquiring survival knowledge, practicing skills, and staying mentally and physically prepared for such situations.

WAR ARTS

In the game of life's battles, let not your size define your might, for the art of deception can turn the tide in the fight. Appear small if you must, but hold a presence vast, for it is through perception that victories are amassed. Like a cunning fox in the shadow, conceal your true form, and let the enemy believe you are a raging storm. Make them doubt, make them question what lies in your wake, and with each step, uncertainty in their hearts you'll make. In subtlety and misdirection, your strength shall reside, For the greatest victories often stem from a well crafted guise. Forge an illusion, a grand spectacle they won't perceive, and watch as they stumble, while you smoothly achieve. Feign weakness when you're strong, let them underestimate, as you quietly prepare to seal their certain fate. In this dance of shadows, let your strategy unfold, and leave your adversaries in a state of wonder. So remember, in this game of wit and art, to feign what you are, and play your role with a cunning heart. For the power lies not in brute force or sheer might, but in the mastery of deception,
Hidden in plain sight.

An adaptation thought derived from The Art of War by Sun Tzu, which I would highly recommend you at least searching this on the Internet long enough to say you might have read it to your friends. It's worth it, and a lot of the takes from it are usable in everyday and big decision time choices.

His Hammer.

She,
His love,
Embraced
With tender grace,
In his heart's chamber,
Her radiant face. Yet creation,
His calling, pulls him deep, While his
Curse of destruction begins to creep.
Love, once cherished, now battles with his
mind, As demons within howl and unwind.
He's torn between passion's gentle song,
And, the chaos that within him throngs.
In his quest to shape worlds with his hands,
Love oft takes second place,
She understands. But through the storm, a
flicker of light,
Love's flame persists,
Burning ever bright.
She,
His muse,
Supports his troubled soul,
Guiding him back to love's gentle fold.
For within the chaos,
Their hearts entwined,
Love's beauty, eternal and refined.

I'm not saying that a person has to have a person in this world, but if you so choose to, make sure it is someone that can withstand yourself, you cannot blame the other person when they can't handle you, it isn't their fault. The storms for some get very dark, and those that understand, understand. At times you just jump into my tornado

in my other is trust

In the realm of trust,

A special bond unfolds, Where hearts are woven, secrets yet untold. An exploration of desires, a delicate art, Two souls entwined, a journey to embark. In this dance of passion, one takes the lead, Guiding with tenderness, Fulfilling each need. A dance of power, a connection profound, Exploring boundaries, on solid ground. With whispers and caresses, they navigate, A symphony of pleasure, a shared fate. In their embrace, vulnerability blooms, A Sanctuary of love, where darkness consumes.

Through tender touch, they ignite the
Flame, In unison they soar,
Their desires untamed.
A partnership of trust,
A sacred connection,
A bond that transcends, defying convention.
They challenge each other to grow and evolve,
Discovering depths, their spirits resolve.
With respect and compassion, they create,
A space of acceptance, where they liberate.
So let us celebrate this journey divine,
Where hearts and
Bodies intertwine.
In this dance of love,
They both find grace,
Embracing desires, in this sacred space.

This means so many things to so many people, and within something so beautiful can also be so often misunderstood, just like Ride or Die."Oh hell yeah I'm your ride or die" But are you? Do you understand? It's a commitment, it's not about if you screw up, it is when. And that is the person that will show up and ride it out. It doesn't matter the fault, because your just there, till my heart stops, some of us walk in the dark and can't come out, and you see me, even when the shadows cover my view.

Dr. Grant's Limb Lab

IN THE HEART OF A BUSTLING METROPOLIS, A HIDDEN LABORATORY THRIVES. DR. ALEXANDER GRANT, THE ECCENTRIC GENIUS BEHIND THE LIMB LAB, IS HERE TO MAKE YOUR WILDEST DREAMS A REALITY. BRACE YOURSELF FOR A THRILLING JOURNEY INTO A WORLD OF EXTRAORDINARY POSSIBILITIES! WITH A WAVE OF HIS HAND, DR. GRANT UNVEILS HIS LATEST CREATIONS: THE GORILLA GRIP AND THE OCTO-ARMS! NEED TO CONQUER ANY PHYSICAL CHALLENGE? THE GORILLA GRIP WILL TRANSFORM YOUR ARMS INTO POWERFUL APPENDAGES, CAPABLE OF FEATS THAT DEFY IMAGINATION. SWING THROUGH TREES, LIFT COLOSSAL WEIGHTS, AND FEEL THE UNTAMED STRENGTH SURGE THROUGH YOUR VEINS. BUT WAIT, THERE'S MORE! INTRODUCING THE OCTO-ARMS, AN INCREDIBLE FUSION OF HUMAN AND CEPHALOPOD INGENUITY. WITH THESE REMARKABLE LIMBS, YOU'LL POSSESS UNPARALLELED DEXTERITY AND MIND-BOGGLING MULTITASKING SKILLS. JUGGLE TASKS EFFORTLESSLY, EXCEL IN PRECISION CRAFTS, AND BECOME THE ULTIMATE PROBLEM-SOLVING MAESTRO. BUT HOW DOES IT WORK, YOU ASK? DR. GRANT'S SECRET LIES IN CUTTING-EDGE ELECTROMAGNETIC TECHNOLOGY. THESE MARVELS OF ENGINEERING SEAMLESSLY LOCK INTO PLACE AT YOUR SHOULDER JOINTS, ALLOWING FOR EFFORTLESS ATTACHMENT AND DETACHMENT. SWAP OUT LIMBS AS EASILY AS CHANGING CLOTHES, ADAPTING TO ANY SITUATION WITH A SIMPLE FLICK OF THE WRIST. BUT IT DOESN'T STOP THERE! THE LIMB LAB OFFERS AN ARRAY OF FANTASTICAL ADD-ONS TO FURTHER AUGMENT YOUR CAPABILITIES. NEED A BOOST IN AGILITY? THE CHEETAH SPRINGS WILL HAVE YOU DARTING THROUGH LIFE WITH LIGHTNING-FAST SPEED. DESIRE ENHANCED VISION? THE EAGLE EYES WILL GRANT YOU A HAWK-LIKE GAZE, SPOTTING DETAILS THAT OTHERS CAN ONLY DREAM OF. AT THE LIMB LAB, WE BELIEVE IN A WORLD WHERE LIMITATIONS ARE SHATTERED, WHERE YOU BECOME THE HERO OF YOUR OWN STORY. STEP INTO OUR REALM OF INNOVATION AND UNLOCK YOUR EXTRAORDINARY POTENTIAL. WITH DR. GRANT AS YOUR GUIDE, PREPARE TO EMBARK ON AN ADVENTURE LIKE NO OTHER. SO, ARE YOU READY TO REDEFINE WHAT IT MEANS TO BE HUMAN? JOIN THE LIMB LAB REVOLUTION TODAY AND LET YOUR IMAGINATION SOAR TO NEW HEIGHTS!

Wonder if he could make me a T-Rex arm? Not like a short stubby little arm but like a T-Rex head and neck just mounted from a little bit back from my wrist. Yes I'm aware of size issues, but come on we can make like toy dog breeds so we can make a toy t-Rex right?

Distant Meadows

In a meadow bright and gold,
Dandelions and secrets they hold
Whispers soft, like lullabies
Inviting dreams under sunny skies
Seeds take flight on gentle breeze
Floating high, like magic keys
Pirouetting in the air, they dance
and twirl, Spreading wishes, like
a precious pearl, Flowers bloom
In vibrant hues
Filling hearts with joy anew
But shadows loom as daylight wanes
Peace disrupted, only chaos remains
Winds cold howl, a somber song
Troubles brew, and hope seems gone
Meadow trembles, fears take hold
In the midst of a story untold
Yet amidst the fear and strife
Seeds of hope will bring new life
With hope and strength, we'll find our way
Rebuilding the meadow, come whatever may
So let us gather, hand in hand
Restore the beauty
Reclaim the land
In unity, we'll mend each part
Healing the meadow
A fresh start
In the meadow's embrace
We find peace true
Amidst the chaos
We'll rise anew.

The sad truth of the world is that things tend to be so tranquil and calm before the first strike of lightning, the first cries often come out of the blue and we are seemingly unprepared, but the best and only thing we can do is accept the world. We accept that we only have the power to control our reaction to exterior events, and not the fact that something has already happened.

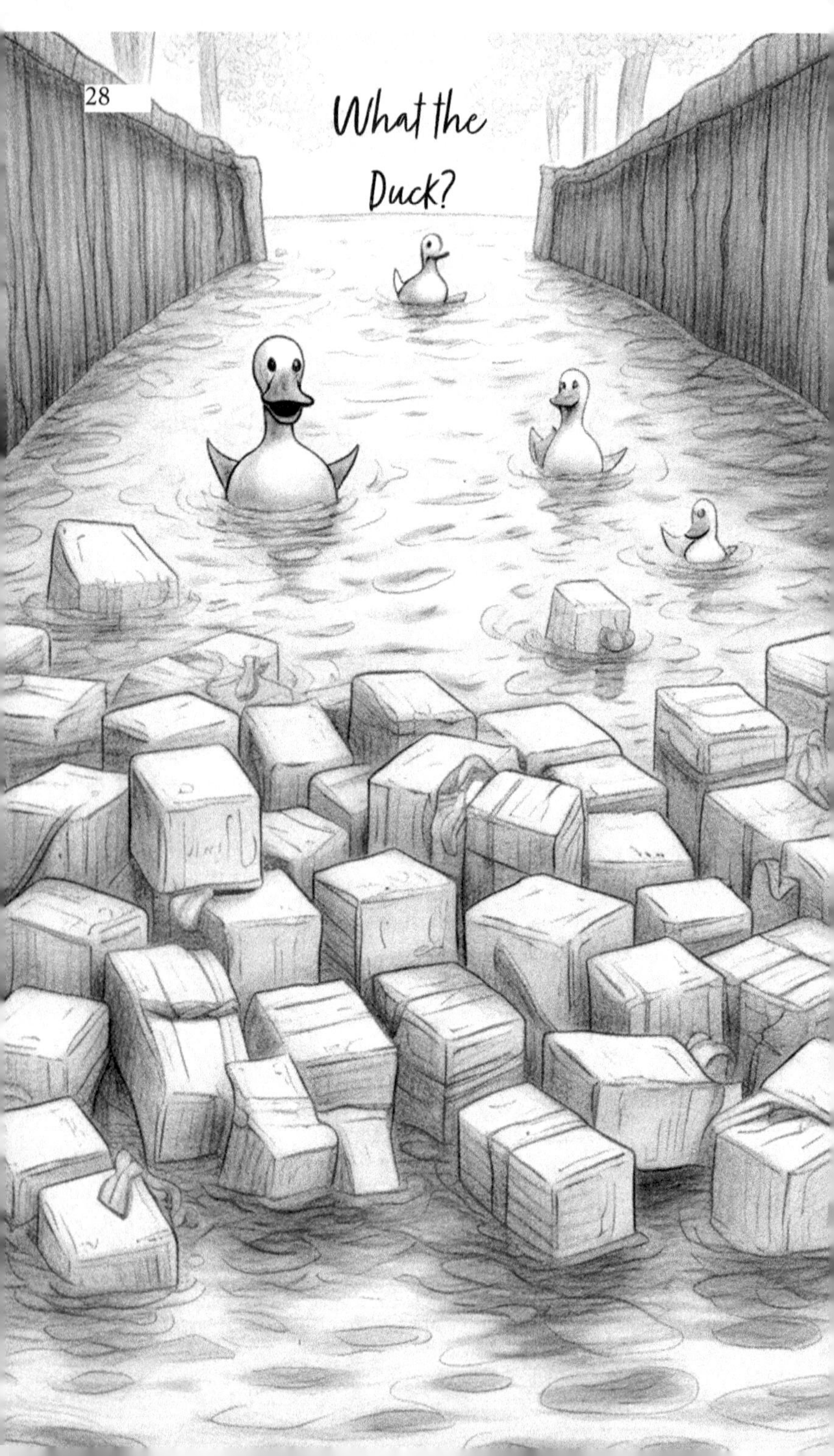

What the
Duck?

EXCERPT FROM MEDITATIONS BY MARCUS AURELIUS

XXIX. Stir up thy mind, and recall thy wits again from thy natural dreams, and visions, and when thou art perfectly awoken, and canst perceive that they were but dreams that troubled thee, as one newly awakened out of another kind of sleep look upon these worldly things with the same mind as thou didst upon those, that thou sawest in thy sleep.

XXX. I consist of body and soul. Unto my body all things are indifferent, for of itself it cannot affect one thing more than another with apprehension of any difference; as for my mind, all things which are not within the verge of her own operation, are indifferent unto her, and for her own operations, those altogether depend of her; neither does she busy herself about any, but those that are present; for as for future and past operations, those also are now at this present indifferent unto her.

XXXI. As long as the foot doth that which belongeth unto it to do, and the hand that which belongs unto it, their labour, whatsoever it be, is not unnatural. So a man as long as he doth that which is proper unto a man, his labour cannot be against nature; and if it be not against nature, then neither is it hurtful unto him. But if it were so that happiness did consist in pleasure: how came notorious robbers, impure abominable livers, parricides, and tyrants, in so large a measure to have their part of pleasures?

XXXII. Dost thou not see, how even those that profess mechanic arts, though in some respect they be no better than mere idiots, yet they stick close to the course of their trade, neither can they find in their heart to decline from it: and is it not a grievous thing that an architect, or a physician shall respect the course and mysteries of their profession, more than a man the proper course and condition of his own nature, reason, which is common to him and to the Gods?

XXXIII. Asia, Europe; what are they, but as corners of the whole world; of which the whole sea, is but as one drop; and the great Mount Athos, but as a clod, as all present time is but as one point of eternity. All, petty things; all things that are soon altered, soon perished. And all things come from one beginning; either all severally and particularly deliberated and resolved upon, by the general ruler and governor of all; or all by necessary consequence. So that the dreadful hiatus of a gaping lion, and all poison, and all hurtful things, are but (as the thorn and the mire) the necessary consequences of goodly fair things. Think not of these therefore, as things contrary to those which thou dost much honour, and respect; but consider in thy mind the true fountain of all.

XXXIV He that seeth the things that are now, hath Seen all that either was ever, or ever shall be, for all things are of one kind; and all like one unto another. Meditate often upon the connection of all things in the world; and upon the mutual relation that they have one unto another. For all things are after a sort folded and involved one within another, and by these means all agree well together. For one thing is consequent unto another, by local motion, by natural conspiration and agreement, and by substantial union, or, reduction of all substances into one.

XXXV. Fit and accommodate thyself to that estate and to those occurrences, which by the destinies have been annexed unto thee; and love those men whom thy fate it is to live with; but love them truly. An instrument, a tool, an utensil, whatsoever it be, if it be fit for the purpose it was made for, it is as it should be though he perchance that made and fitted it, be out of sight and gone. But in things natural, that power which hath framed and fitted them, is and abideth within them still: for which reason she ought also the more to be respected, and we are the more obliged (if we may live and pass our time according to her purpose and intention) to think that all is well with us, and according to our own minds. After this manner also, and in this respect it is, that he that is all in all doth enjoy his happiness.

Though I do not wholly embrace all of the school of Stoicism I do look upon Marcus Aurelius in moments that I need some thought guidance, or to handle a situation. It became one of the base foundations along with Art of War at a young age to help me develop my masking skills to blend in with those around me. It humbled me and helped to shape my always smiling persona, it isn't always the healthiest mentally but at times survival is king.

MENTAL RIDDLES

I can weigh heavily on your mind yet I'm invisible to the eye. When you share me I become lighter. What am I?
~~Problem~~

I am a prison without walls, where the captives are trapped in their own thoughts. What am I?
~~Anxiety~~

I can bring both joy and sorrow, and at times, I may feel like an endless battle. Some embrace me, while others fear me. What am I?
~~Emotion~~

I am a thief that steals your peace, leaving you restless and tired. I invade your nights, but disappear in the morning light. What am I?
~~Insomnia~~

I am a maze of distorted thoughts, a realm where reality gets distorted and caught. I whisper lies and sow seeds of doubt, but therapy and self-care can help you break out. What am I?
~~Paranoia~~

I'm a shroud that covers your sunny days, casting a shadow on life's joyful rays. I drain your energy and dampen your zest, but with self-compassion, you can find rest. What am I?
~~Fatigue~~

I'm sometimes upside down, sometimes right-side up, and when you sit I get kinda stuck. What am I?
I could be your butt.

UNEXPLORED PLACES

In realms unseen,
Where shadows dance,An enigma awaits,
A mystic trance.
Whispers of secrets, whispered low,
Unraveling truths
We yearn to know.
Minds in motion, thoughts untamed,
In the depths of chaos,
They're unchained. The flicker of madness,
A kaleidoscope show,
Where sanity falters, and visions glow.
Through twists and turns,
They ebb and flow,
Creatures of the mind, come and go.
In the tapestry of thoughts,
They sow,
A symphony of madness, a riddle to bestow.
By the edge of reason,
Where edges blur,
The enigma of the mind begins to stir.
Exploring depths where
Few dare to tread,
A journey within, where worlds are spread.
So embrace
The unknown,
Embrace the wild,
For in the chaos, creativity is beguiled.
In the realm of madness,
Truths may lie,
Stare into the void deep,
Using vision beyond your eyes.

Sometimes that which we know and that which we do not, run along a razors edge, but the thing about the edge of the razor isn't how close things are at the start, but by the descent they are worlds apart. So is that which we do not know, it's impossible to know just how different something or someone can be.

RIVER OF MIND

In twilight's gentle glow,
By the riverside I stand,
Where roaring waters rush, as if by Nature's command.
The evening sun retreats, casting a golden hue,
And the moon, serene and bright, hangs in the sky so blue.
But as I gaze upon this scene, a river in my mind,Thoughts cascade like
waterfalls, a tumultuous bind. The currents twist and turn, a torrent
of confusion, Whispering voices rise, a chaotic fusion. I see the moon's
reflection dancing on the restless waves, A fragmented reflection of the
thoughts my mind engraves. The beauty of the scene, with a haunting
undertone, As sanity and madness intertwine, a world unknown. The
gentle lapping of the waves, a rhythmic melody,
Yet within my troubled mind, a cacophony of frenzy.
The moon's steady glow, a beacon in the night, But my thoughts, like
wayward stars, refuse to align, take flight. Oh, how I long to find solace in
this tranquil sight, To tame the raging river, bring order to the night. But
as the river flows, I must navigate its course, A journey through the tempest, seeking inner force. For within this chaotic river, a soul yearns to be
 heard, A tale of strength and resilience, like the flight of a bird. Though
My mind may be a maze, with twists and turns untold,I'll strive to find my
Way, and embrace the stories yet unfold. So let me walk beside this river,
With hope as my guide, Through the ebb and flow of life, where peace
May reside. In the depths of my being, a flicker of light will gleam,
A reminder that I'm more than the chaos within my dream.
And as the evening sun dips, and the moon takes its reign,
I'll embrace the beauty and the darkness, without refrain.
For within this ever-changing river, my spirit will strive,
To find harmony and grace,
As I navigate this life.

I go back to the river concept a lot, mostly because it seems at times the best fitting,
something between that and the feeling of floating at the bottom of the deep end of a pool.
Pressure on top of pressure until you feel like the kettle on the stove about to scream.

LOST IN THOUGHTS

In the
Labyrinthine
Recesses of a
Shattered mind,
Thoughts   tangle
Like unruly   vines, weaving
A tapestry   of fragmented
Whispers and   muffled cries. A
Kaleidoscope   of emotions dances in
Disarray, colors bleeding   into one another,
A chaotic symphony of   shattered dreams. Words
stumble and falter,   lost in the labyrinth of
Fractured memories,   as sanity's delicate
Thread unravels,   unraveling the fabric
Of reality itself.   Shadows cast by
Phantom fears   morph into
Grotesque specters,   haunting the
Corridors of thought,   while fractured
Mirrors reflect   fractured souls,
Reflecting an   internal landscape,
Fractured and   raw. Echoes of
Forgotten   melodies linger,
Intermingling with   the dissonance
Of discordant   thoughts, a symphony
Of discord woven   into the very fabric of
Existence. Yet, amidst   the chaos, glimmers
Of ethereal beauty emerge,   like fragile
stars against the backdrop of   darkness, illu-
minating
The intricate tapestry   of a broken mind.

Sometimes the best thing we can do is put a face on while we process, allow the mask to do its job while we determine how to best pursue something, whether we are stuck looking at the game aisle in a store, where we periodically get lost for hours thinking of other worlds. Or trying to perform a life saving operation on a patient, I know they seem kinda different but are they really? Both require a level of skill and luck, I mean how many brain surgeons can toss a tomahawk over two city blocks and eliminate the guy camping on the spawn pad?

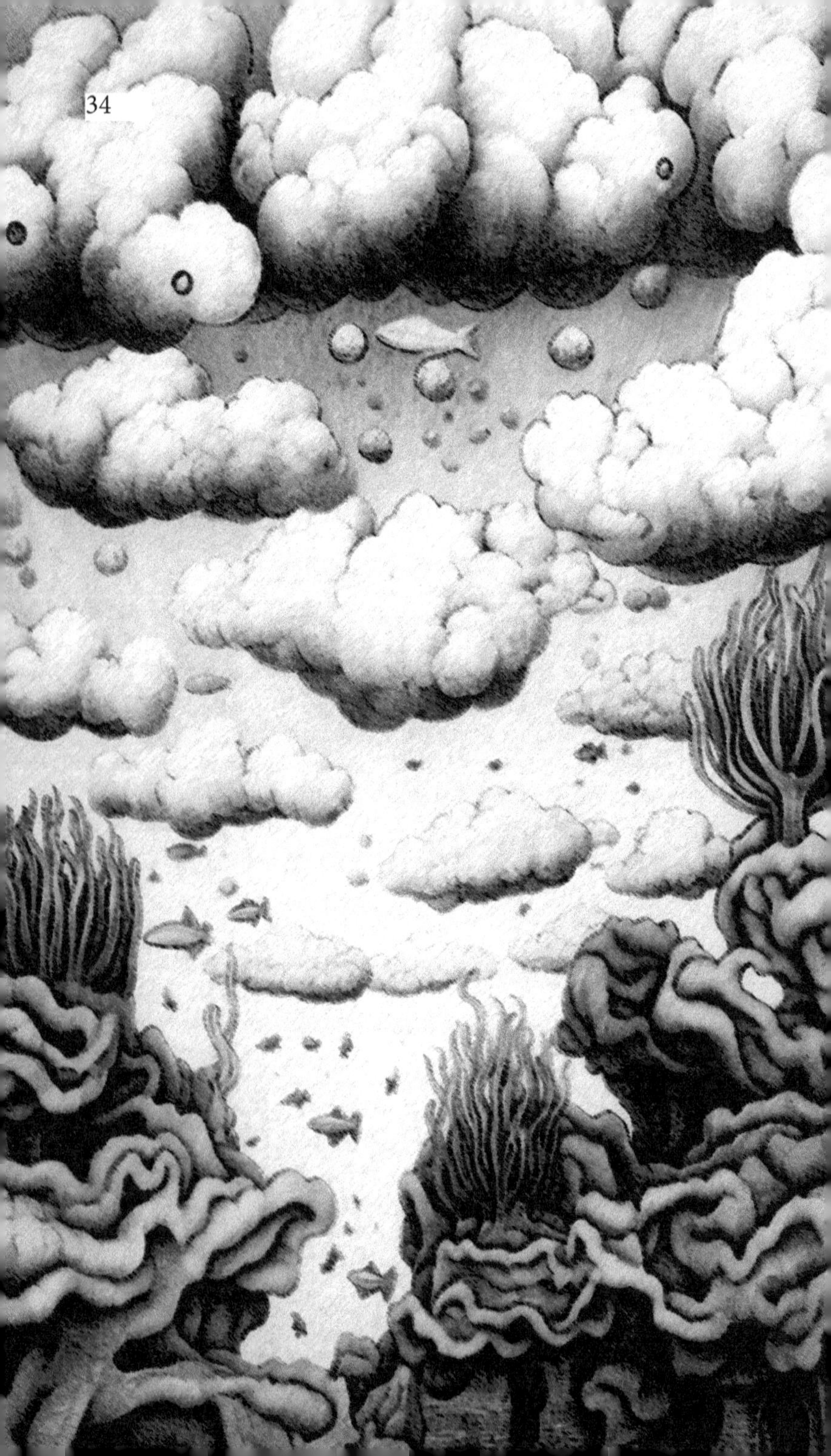

Tanka Timez

Beneath their shadows
I find my hidden fortress
Unleashing my voice
Defying expectations
I rise, a phoenix reborn

In whispers they speak
Labels, chained conformity
But within my heart
Unveiling my true colors
I paint my own masterpiece

I shed their judgments
Embracing my authenticity
Unapologetic
A kaleidoscope of dreams
I dance to my own rhythm

Their eyes may linger
Trying to shape my narrative
Yet I stand steadfast
Writing my own destiny
Inscribed with courage and grace

A tapestry woven
Threads of defiance and hope
I break free, unbound
No longer defined by them
I embrace my true essence

We are often hardest on ourselves then the rest of the world, and this is how it should be, but make sure that you properly direct your energy. Be who you want, picture the image of the you, that you want to be and pour your energy into that. Allow yourself this, please. Think about it, you work hours a day for someone else, do things every day for other people, and this is all okay, just don't lose who you are in what the world wants you to be.

THE ROAD LESS...MORE FORSAKEN.

In a world engulfed by shadows deep,
A path obscured,
Where nightmares creep.
Not the road less traveled,
But forsaken,
Where sanity's grip is
Tattered and shaken.
The beaten path lies
Tranquil and serene,
While the unknown road
Conceals the obscene.
Tread not with caution,
But trepidation,For what awaits
Defies all explanation.
Step forth, into the twisted abyss,
Where choices made ignite a fiery hiss.
The road less traveled, a haunted maze
Where darkness thrives, in dreadful haze.
The footprints left on this forsaken trail,
Echo screams of those who dared to fail.
Their souls consumed by relentless strife,
Lost to the horrors of a twisted life.
The road beckons, with its siren's call,
A haunting invitation, a destined fall.
Choose wisely, for the path's a guise,
Where the road less
Traveled breeds demise.
But should you venture
Into the unknown,
Prepare for the darkness
To claim its own.
For the road less traveled,
A treacherous dance,
Where salvation fades,
And nightmares advance.

Some things in this world require something more then simply seeing,
but for those that have walked in the dark, it marks you... Simple as
that, we can recognize our own

Lightning In a Bottle

He sits at his desk, pen in hand,
A restless mind, aching to expand.
A flood of thoughts,
A rushing stream, endless ideas, each one a dream.
He reaches out, grasping for one, to bring to life, to be undone.
But they slip away, out of his hold,
A sea of thoughts, a story untold.
Days and nights, they blur and blend, As he seeks a way to transcend
The chaos of his racing mind, To a place of calm, a peace to find.
And then he creates, and time stands still, As he paints and composes, with heart and skill. The world fades away,
And he is free,
Lost in the beauty of his own reverie.
But when he stops, the world comes crashing back,
A brutal reality, an unrelenting attack.
His mind races on, a ceaseless tide, An endless storm, he cannot hide.
He longs for peace, a respite from the storm, A moment of quiet, a chance to reform. But his mind roars on, a force to be reckoned,
A powerful surge, a wild reckoning.
He fights and he struggles, but it's all in vain, As his mind takes hold, and drives him insane. A victim of his own limitless imagination, A brilliant mind, trapped in its own damnation. And so he lives, a tortured soul, A victim of a mind he cannot control.
But in his art, a legacy is born, a testament to the beauty he has adorned.

I originally felt so... gross putting this in the book, it seems so personal and woe is me, until I start to think of the other people out there that might feel the same way... and sometimes it's the one person reading the right thing that changes a life. I guess.

Surviving a Flaming Tornado on a Hydrogen Blimp?
Strictly just some common sense, don't sue me if it happens and you drop your sunglasses off the side.

Take Immediate Action: Stay calm and assess the situation quickly. Activate any emergency systems or alarms on the blimp.

Protect Yourself: Find a secure location on the blimp away from flames and potential hazards. Use any available fire-resistant materials to shield yourself from the heat.

Communication: Establish communication with the blimp's crew and passengers. Inform them about the situation and coordinate a response plan.

Emergency Equipment: Locate and use any available fire extinguishers or fire suppression systems. Equip yourself with a fire-resistant suit if available.

Seek Shelter: Identify areas on the blimp that offer increased protection from the flames. Move towards enclosed spaces, such as cabins or compartments.

Evacuation: If the blimp is at a safe altitude and the situation is uncontrollable, consider an emergency evacuation plan. Utilize available parachutes or escape pods if provided.

Descending Safely: If forced to descend, aim for an area away from populated areas, structures, and other potential hazards. Look for open fields or bodies of water as potential landing spots.

Impact Preparation: Brace for impact by assuming a protective position and securing loose objects. Use any available cushions or padding to minimize injuries upon landing.

Post-Landing Actions: Once on the ground, move away from the blimp and the flaming tornado to a safe distance. Assess injuries and provide immediate first aid to yourself and others if needed.

Seek Help: Contact emergency services or alert nearby individuals about the situation. Follow any specific emergency protocols or procedures for reporting the incident.

I mean... We all know at least half of the people on the blimp are going to be live streaming the whole thing and the other half will be watching it on their phones instead right? So maybe remember to grab the little bungee band that you put on the arms of your sunglasses and they won't fall off.

Parental Anxieties

With anticipation I watch him grow, with my heart I think I know. Within his self are parts of me, my prismatic imperfections for him to be The things that make me struggle, the things that I don't know, in this world we do as we can, the things we think work, and try to make little plans. I know from past that future is a crap shot with busted gamblers knees. Have I done enough to prepare him, did I do what I thought was right? Did I let him cry to long by himself in the night? Do they learn from what we do or from the things that we can teach? Will he carry my bad habits, will he shepherd in his lost mind? Can the things that I've thought somehow break him? Is the water to hot or cold for his skin? The questions seems to grow and answers go to and fro, you never know what your going to get until you sit and listen to the symphony, the falling motif setting the stage and preparing your the build into the first verse, seemingly taking you along and showing you the worst parts of yourself that you never wanted him to pick up, and then as you again fade back into that old few notes signaling that soon you will once again be at the stage in life that something else grows, something else changes and you have to ask yourself a million more questions, and they are smiling as your anxiety has convinced you that you have created a serial killer because he dunked one of his rubber ducks in the tub and laughed about it... But I mean that's how it starts right?

This section is pretty self explanatory I mean we do what we can, the best we can, sometimes shit happens and we get some scars, and hopefully that's the worse, we all know that it isn't as bad is it gets... but for a light hearted yet attempt at random insightful book geared towards young adults... well it's as rough as it needs to get.

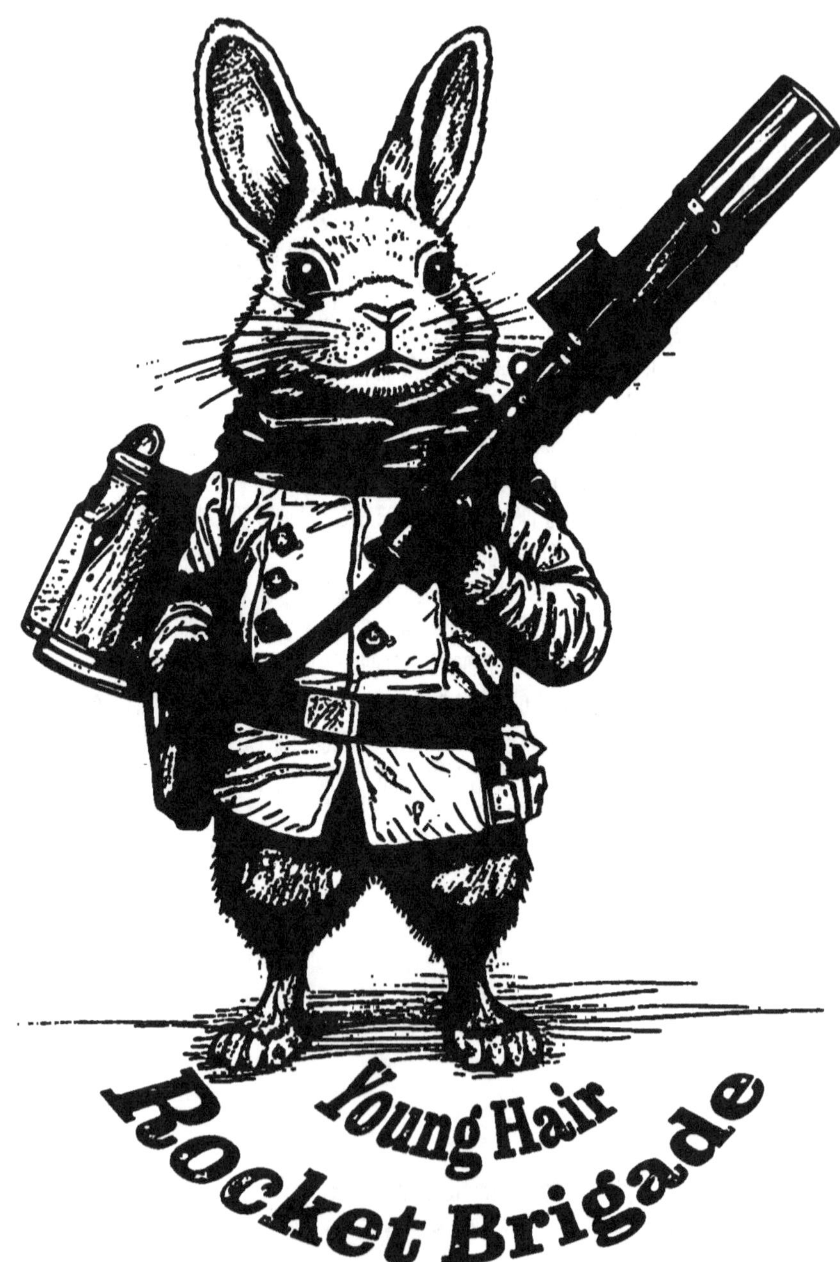

Young Hair
Rocket Brigade

Who will they be?

She
Sits alone
No place like home
She sits and thinks
Hasn't slept right in weeks
Still stuck in her head it's constant
Dread can't seem to get ahead
She writes down her last thoughts
Simple things that she thinks she thought
Little words that seemed to sum up the last plot
Little birds she set free so maybe the world
They could see, maybe they could learn to fly
Maybe they could be, something she never could
Be, something that was bigger then itself
Something that was truly for all the yous
Beyond the mes, something that would share
For the world to see, to grow, to love, to create
But how can you teach love when you only
Know it because your heart beats?
How can you teach to feel when you yourself can't
Find the words to bleed
Or the right thoughts to seed
How can I teach him when I haven't yet found my wings? How
can he fly if I'm afraid to be me.
What mirror can I show him when I simply
Copy what I see? What kinda life can he
Ever hope to have when I can't be
What he needs, give him a home
But the home needs heat
Give him the shirt off my back
Still need a bed to sleep
Everything for everyone that needs
A parents head can be a mess indeed.

This is just so relatable from different positions, different head spaces, I have a family history of... Self elimination and the attempting of such. It's no stranger to my own mind, it's nothing personal, it's hard to take it any way but though. It's like a backpack though and you put everything in it and start, and find something and grab it, and find something and grab it, and before you know it... well it's full and your tired. We can only collect so much.

Surviving a Fog of invisibility?
Strictly just some common sense, don't sue me if it happens and you break your arm patting yourself on the back right before an invisible tiger eats you.

Move with Caution: As you become invisible in the fog, exercise extreme care when walking or running. Although you may feel protected, remember that you are still susceptible to injury from obstacles such as fallen branches, hidden pits, or uneven terrain. Proceed slowly and deliberately to avoid accidents.

Use Sound as a Guide: In this fog, visibility is compromised, but your presence can still be detected through sound. Utilize sound as a way to communicate with others in your group and establish a system of auditory signals to stay connected and avoid accidental separation.

Create Auditory Distractions: Take advantage of the fog's property by generating sound to divert the attention of potential threats. Throw pebbles, snap twigs, or use other objects to create noise in a different direction, drawing attention away from your actual location.

Employ Scent-Masking Techniques: While invisible, you may still emit scents that animals can detect. To minimize the risk of attracting unwanted attention, familiarize yourself with natural scents in the environment and employ techniques such as rubbing foliage on your clothing or applying mud to your body to mask your scent.

Seek Higher Ground: As the unseen fog tends to settle closer to the ground, ascending to higher elevations can help you gain a clearer view of your surroundings. Climbing trees or finding elevated terrain can offer a vantage point to assess the area and plan your next move.

Carry Lightweight Noisemakers: To enhance your ability to create sounds when needed, equip yourself with lightweight, compact noisemakers. Whistles, small bells, or even jingling keys can serve as effective tools for attracting attention or signaling for help.

Stay Alert and Listen: Since visibility is limited, rely on your other senses. Train your ears to pick up subtle sounds and movements in the environment. Listen for rustling leaves, breaking twigs, or the faintest animal calls, as these may indicate the presence of potential threats or nearby sources of help.

If I had a tree for every time I ran into one I would have 3 trees... and they each would get cut down cause it hurts. Fog seems like it would make my clumsy ass fly into something, off of something, and then into something, hopefully not something with sharp teeth.. or magma.

* 9 7 9 8 2 1 8 2 3 0 7 1 5 *